Comprehensive lipid testing and management

Comprehensive lipid testing and management

Lars A Carlson
King Gustaf V Research Institute
Karolinska Institutet
Stockholm, Sweden

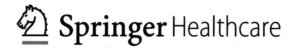 Springer Healthcare

Published by Springer Healthcare Ltd, 236 Gray's Inn Road, London, WC1X 8HL, UK.

www.springerhealthcare.com

British Library Cataloguing-in-Publication Data.

A catalogue record for this book is available from the British Library.

ISBN 978-1-907673-03-0

Although every effort has been made to ensure that drug doses and other information are presented accurately in this publication, the ultimate responsibility rests with the prescribing physician. Neither the publisher nor the authors can be held responsible for errors or for any consequences arising from the use of the information contained herein. Any product mentioned in this publication should be used in accordance with the prescribing information prepared by the manufacturers. No claims or endorsements are made for any drug or compound at present under clinical investigation.

Commissioning editor: Ian Stoneham

Project editor: Alison Whitehouse and Tamsin Curtis

Designer: Joe Harvey

Artworker: Sissan Mollerfors

Production: Marina Maher

Contents

Author biography

Professor Lars A Carlson is currently Emeritus Research Professor at the Karolinska Institutet and Director of the Lipid and Hypertension Clinic at Sophiahemmet, Stockholm, Sweden. He qualified in medicine at the Karolinska Institutet, and later obtained his PhD there. His clinical training was undertaken at the Department of Internal Medicine, Karolinska Hospital. He became the first Swedish Professor of Geriatric Medicine in Uppsala and created the Department of Geriatric Medicine at Uppsala University. This was followed by positions at the Karolinska Institutet as Professor of Internal Medicine and at the Department of Internal Medicine, Karolinska Hospital as a Consultant Physician. At the same time he was Director of the King Gustaf V Research Institute, Karolinska Institutet. He has also been a Visiting Professor at the Royal Postgraduate Medical School, Hammersmith Hospital, London, and the University Department of Medicine, Hopital Cantonal, Geneva, Switzerland.

Professor Carlson has been the President of the European Society for Clinical Investigation and the European Atherosclerosis Society. He has been the editor of the journal *Atherosclerosis* and has published some 500 scientific articles. For 20 years he has been a member of the Nobel Assembly, Karolinska Institutet. His main research interests include clinical lipidology and atherosclerosis. He received the prestigious Oscar Minkowski Prize of the European Diabetes Society and several other national and international awards for scientific achievements.

Abbreviations

ACCORD	Action to Control Cardiovascular Risk in Diabetes
AIM-HIGH	The Atherothrombosis Intervention in Metabolic Syndrome with Low HDL-C/High Triglyceride and Impact on Global Health Outcomes
AMORIS	Apolipoprotein Related Mortality Risk Study
ARBITER	Arterial Biology for the Investigation of the Treatment Effects of Reducing Cholesterol
ARBITER 6-HALTS	Arterial Biology for the Investigation of the Treatment Effects of Reducing Cholesterol 6 – HDL and LDL Treatment Strategies
ATP III	Third Report of the Expert Panel on Detection, Evaluation, and Treatment of High Blood Cholesterol in Adults
BIP	Bezafibrate Infarction Prevention trial
CARDS	Collaborative Atorvastatin Diabetes Study
CDPP	community diabetes prevention project
CDP	Coronary Drug Project
CIMT	carotid intima-media thickness
CPPT	Coronary Primary Prevention Trial
CTT	Cholesterol Treatment Trialists
DAIS	Diabetes Atherosclerosis Intervention Study
ENHANCE	Ezetimibe and Simvastatin in Hypercholesterolemia Enhances Atherosclerosis Regression
FIELD	Fenofibrate Intervention and Event Lowering in Diabetes
HDL, HDL2, HDL3	high-density lipoprotein
HATS	HDL Atherosclerosis Treatment Study
HHS	Helsinki Heart Study
HPS	Heart Protection Study
HPS2-THRIVE	HPS 2: Treatment of HDL to Reduce the Incidence of Vascular Events

IMPROVE-IT	Improved Reduction of Outcomes: Vytorin Efficacy International Trial
LDL	low-density lipoprotein
Lp(a)	lipoprotein (a)
MPT	microsomal triglyceride transfer protein
NCEP	National Cholesterol Education Program
4S	Scandinavian Simvastatin Survival Study
SANDS	Stop Atherosclerosis in Native Diabetics Study
SEAS	Simvastatin and Ezetimibe in Aortic Stenosis trial
SHARP	Study of Heart and Renal Protection
STELLAR	Statin Therapies for Elevated Lipid Levels Compared Across Doses to Rosuvastatin
TLC	therapeutic lifestyle change
TNT	Treat to New Target
VA-HIT	Veterans Affairs High-Density Lipoprotein Intervention Trial
VLDL	very low-density lipoprotein

PART ONE

Lipid testing

Chapter 1

Atherosclerosis and clinical atherosclerosis

Atherosclerosis

Atherosclerotic cardiovascular diseases are the major cause of mortality for both men and women in the industrial as well as the developing world, with the majority of deaths occurring in developing countries [1,2]. In addition, diseases due to atherosclerosis such as coronary artery disease (CAD) causing coronary heart disease (CHD), cerebrovascular diseases and peripheral vascular diseases which here are called clinical atherosclerosis, cause considerable morbidity and disability. The major manifestations of clinical atherosclerosis are listed in Figure 1.1.

Atherosclerosis, now believed to be an inflammatory disease [3], begins with an accumulation of cholesterol rich low-density lipoproteins in the arterial intima. Subsequently a number of immunological processes take place, culminating with formation of lipid-loaded foam cells, growing atherosclerotic plaques, narrowing of the arteries, plaque rupture, thrombus formation, ischaemia and infarction and other manifestations of clinical atherosclerosis [3].

Risk factors for clinical atherosclerosis

The term 'risk factor' comprises factors which, if present, are associated with an increased risk for a specific disease. The 'risk factor' concept emerged for the first time in a lecture given by Doyle in 1963 in a meeting at the Medical Society of the State of New York [4]. Doyle presented results from a 10-year follow up of 2000 men in Albany, New York, showing that high values of cholesterol and blood pressure, as well as smoking were associated with the occurrence of CHD and were therefore

Manifestations of clinical atherosclerosis	
Coronary heart disease	• Sudden death
	• Myocardial infarction (acute coronary syndromes)
	• Unstable angina
	• Angina pectoris
Cerebrovascular disease	• Transitory ischaemic attacks
	• Cerebral infarction (stroke)
Atherosclerotic peripheral vascular disease	• Intermittent claudication
	• Critical limb ischaemia leading to tissue death

Figure 1.1 Manifestations of clinical atherosclerosis.

risk factors. The full emergence for the risk factor concept in relation to clinical atherosclerosis came, however, around 1960 with the report by the Framingham Heart Study, 'Factors of risk in the development of coronary heart disease' [5].

It is noteworthy that a risk factor is not necessarily causative for the disease and may only be an *associated* phenomenon – a risk marker. For a risk factor to be causative it is required that it is present before the disease occurs and that the causality is biologically reasonable. Furthermore, if the specific treatment or removal of a risk factor – such as reduction of a high cholesterol level or cessation of smoking – leads to a reduced risk, this would support causality.

A risk factor can be numerical, for example cholesterol level and blood pressure, or categorical, for example gender and smoking habit.

Traditional risk factors

For both prevention and treatment of clinical atherosclerosis, the identification and diagnosis of those causative risk factors that are amendable is of the greatest importance. Case–control studies as well as prospective studies have documented a number of risk factors for clinical atherosclerosis.

The most common and generally accepted major risk factors for clinical atherosclerosis are given in Figure 1.2, in which they are classified as either 'modifiable' or 'non-modifiable'. Controlled clinical trials have shown that treatment of modifiable lipid risk factors by therapeutic lifestyle changes (TLCs, e.g. improvement of diet, smoking cessation and increased physical activity) or by pharmacological means (with statins in the forefront, followed by fibrates and nicotinic acid) reduces the occurrence of manifestations of clinical atherosclerosis.

The global risk factor panorama from the INTERHEART study

Most studies establishing the various risk factors for atherosclerosis have been done in Europe and the USA. It is not certain to what extent these findings are valid globally. There is clear evidence that the risk factor panorama may vary between populations. For example, hypertension may be more important as a risk factor in Japan and China than it is in Europe and the USA, while lipid levels may be less important risk factors for clinical atherosclerosis in south Asia than in many other regions in the world.

The recently published large INTERHEART studies [6,7] were designed to assess the importance of risk factors for CHD worldwide. The study was conducted in 52 countries representing every inhabited continent and comprised 15,152 cases of recent myocardial infarction and 14,820 age-matched controls.

Nine global risk factors for myocardial infarction that emerged from the INTERHEART study in all regions, at all ages and in both sexes are presented in Figure 1.3.

Results for lipids and lipoproteins are dealt with below [7]. When combined, these nine risk factors accounted for about 90% of the

Classic major risk factors for clinical atherosclerosis	
Modifiable	**Nonmodifiable**
Dyslipidaemia (high LDL, low HDL, high triglycerides)	Age
Hypertension	Male gender
Smoking	Manifestations of clinical atherosclerosis
Diabetes/insulin resistance	Family history of coronary heart disease
Obesity	Menopause
Metabolic syndrome	
Physical inactivity	

Figure 1.2 The classic major risk factors for clinical atherosclerosis. This is the risk factor panorama that has been evolved from case/control and prospective studies in Europe and USA during the latter part of the 20th century. HDL, high-density lipoprotein; LDL, low-density lipoprotein.

population attributable risk (PAR). The PAR values in ranking order for the different risk factors were:

- apolipoprotein B/apolipoprotein A-I (apoB/apoA-I; see below) 49%,
- smoking 36%,
- psychosocial factors 33%,
- abdominal obesity 20%,
- hypertension 18%,
- physical activity 12%, and
- diabetes 10%.

The finding that so many identical items were significant risk factors for myocardial infarction in all the regions studied suggests that similar approaches for the prevention of myocardial infarction may be effective globally.

The quantitative relationship between the two most important risk factors (cigarette smoking and the apoB/apoA-I ratio) and the odds of myocardial infarction are shown in Figure 1.4. Worldwide there is a striking linear increase in risk for myocardial infarction with the number of cigarettes smoked as well as with increasing apoB/apoA-I ratio.

The odds ratios for the nine significant global risk factors for myocardial infarction in the INTERHEART study are given in Figure 1.5. A highly significant risk was associated with smoking, diabetes, hypertension, abdominal obesity, the apoB/apoA-I ratio and psychosocial factors. The data in the figure also suggest the existence of a protective effect from consumption of fruit, exercise and alcohol.

Major global risk factors for myocardial infarction

- Dyslipidaemia
- Smoking
- Hypertension
- Diabetes
- Abdominal obesity
- Psychosocial factors
- Lack of daily consumption of fruits and vegetables
- Lack of regular physical activity
- Alcohol

Figure 1.3 Major global risk factors for myocardial infarction. The global risk factors that emerged in the INTERHEART study [6].

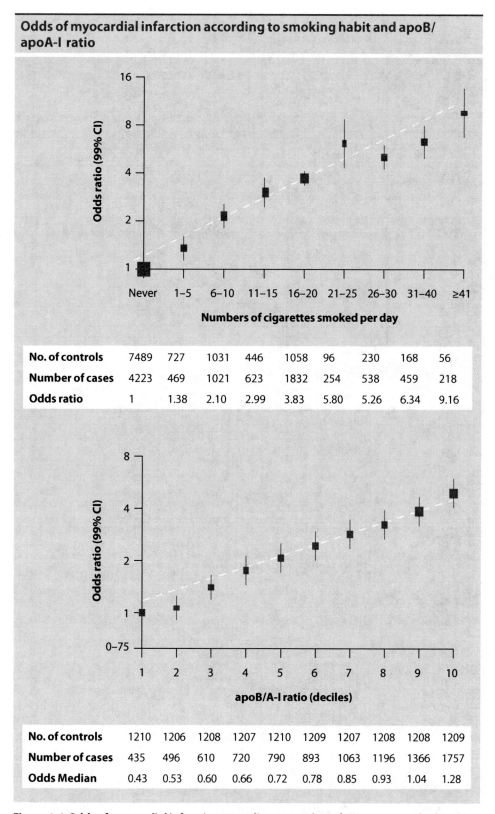

Odds of myocardial infarction according to smoking habit and apoB/apoA-I ratio

No. of controls	7489	727	1031	446	1058	96	230	168	56
Number of cases	4223	469	1021	623	1832	254	538	459	218
Odds ratio	1	1.38	2.10	2.99	3.83	5.80	5.26	6.34	9.16

No. of controls	1210	1206	1208	1207	1210	1209	1207	1208	1208	1209
Number of cases	435	496	610	720	790	893	1063	1196	1366	1757
Odds Median	0.43	0.53	0.60	0.66	0.72	0.78	0.85	0.93	1.04	1.28

Figure 1.4 Odds of myocardial infarction according to number of cigarettes smoked and apoB/apoA-I ratio. Note the log scale on the y axis for both figures. apo, apolipoprotein; CI, confidence interval. Reproduced with permission from Yusuf S et al. Lancet 2004;364:937–952.

Association of risk factors with acute myocardial infarction

Risk factor	Sex	Control (%)	Case (%)	Odds ratio (99% CI)	PAR (99% CI)
Current smoking	F	9.3	20.1	2.86 (2.36–3.48)	15.8% (12.9–19.3)
	M	33.0	53.1	3.05 (2.78–3.33)	44.0% (40.9–47.2)
Diabetes	F	7.9	25.5	4.26 (3.51–5.18)	19.1% (16.8–21.7)
	M	7.4	16.2	2.67 (2.36–3.02)	10.1% (8.9–11.4)
Hypertension	F	28.3	53.0	2.95 (2.57–3.39)	35.8% (32.1–39.6)
	M	19.7	34.6	2.32 (2.12–2.53)	19.5% (17.7–21.5)
Abdominal obesity	F	33.3	45.6	2.26 (1.90–2.68)	35.9% (28.9–43.6)
	M	33.3	46.5	2.24 (2.03–2.47)	32.1% (28.0–36.5)
Psychosocial index	F	–	–	3.49 (2.41–5.04)	40.0% (28.6–52.6)
	M	–	–	2.58 (2.11–3.14)	25.3% (18.2–34.0)
Fruits/veg	F	50.3	39.4	0.58 (0.48–0.71)	17.8% (12.9–24.1)
	M	39.6	34.7	0.74 (0.66–0.83)	10.3% (6.9–15.2)
Exercise	F	16.5	9.3	0.48 (0.39–0.59)	37.3% (26.1–50.0)
	M	20.3	15.8	0.77 (0.69–0.85)	22.9% (16.9–30.2)
Alcohol	F	11.2	6.3	0.41 (0.32–0.53)	46.9% (34.3–60.0)
	M	29.1	29.6	0.88 (0.81–0.96)	10.5% (6.1–17.5)
apoB/apoA-I ratio	F	14.1	27.0	4.42 (3.43–5.70)	52.1% (44.0–60.2)
	M	21.9	35.5	3.76 (3.23–4.38)	53.8% (48.3–59.2)

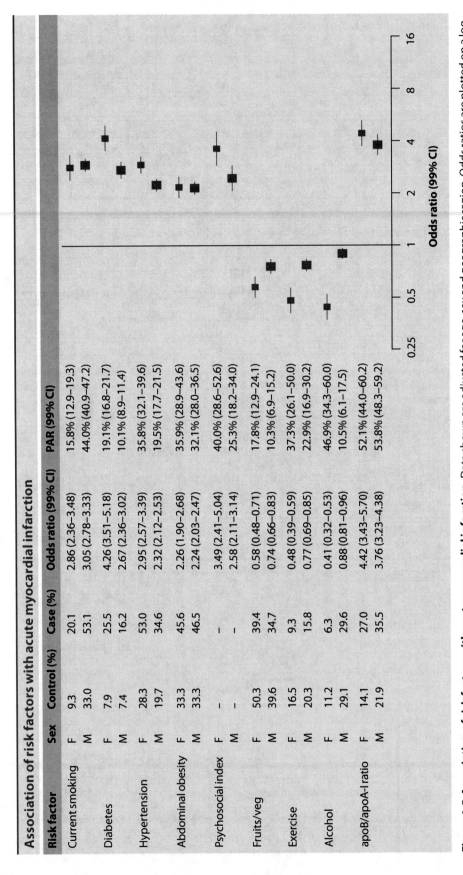

Odds ratio (99% CI)

Figure 1.5 Association of risk factors with acute myocardial infarction. Data shown are adjusted for age, sex and geographic region. Odds ratios are plotted on a log scale. Prevalence cannot be calculated for psychosocial factors because it is derived from a model. apo, apolipoprotein; CI, confidence interval; F, female; M, male; PAR, population-attributable risk. Reproduced with permission from Yusuf S et al. Lancet 2004;364:937–952.

Manifestations of clinical atherosclerosis		
Lipids and lipoproteins	**Lipoprotein subfractions**	**Apolipoproteins**
Cholesterol	Small, dense LDL	apoB
Triglycerides	Oxidised LDL	Low apoA-I
LDL-C		
apoB:apoA-I ratio		
Low HDL-C		
Cholesterol:HDL-C ratio		
LDL-C:HDL-C ratio		
Non-HDL-C		
Lp(a)		

Figure 1.6 Major lipid-related risk factors for clinical atherosclerosis. apo, apolipoprotein; C, cholesterol; HDL, high-density lipoprotein; LDL, low-density lipoprotein; Lp(a), lipoprotein (a).

Lipid-related risk factors for clinical atherosclerosis

The major lipid-related risk factors for clinical atherosclerosis are given in Figure 1.6, and methods for measuring them are described in Chapter 4. The relation between these risk factors and the risk for clinical atherosclerosis is continuous, without discrete threshold values, which is of importance in treatment considerations.

The strong, positive curvilinear relationship between total cholesterol (total-C, representing low-density lipoprotein cholesterol [LDL-C]) and the risk for CHD observed in three large prospective US studies, including the Framingham study, is shown in Figure 1.7. A positive relationship between values for fasting triglycerides and the incidence of myocardial infarction was presented in the Stockholm prospective study (Figure 1.8) and has subsequently been seen in several other studies. For high-density lipoprotein (HDL), in contrast, the Framingham study showed that there was a negative relationship with occurrence of CHD (Figure 1.9); this has been confirmed in many studies and is an indication of the protective role of HDL against CHD.

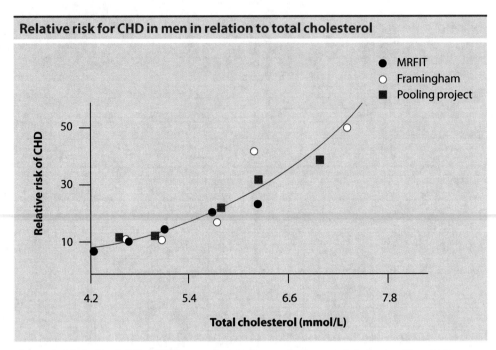

Figure 1.7 Relative risk for CHD in men in relation to plasma total cholesterol levels. Data from three large US studies. CHD, coronary heart disease; MRFIT, Multiple Risk Factor Intervention Trial. Adapted with permission from Klippel JH et al. Internal Medicine, 5th edition. St Louis: Mosby; 1998.

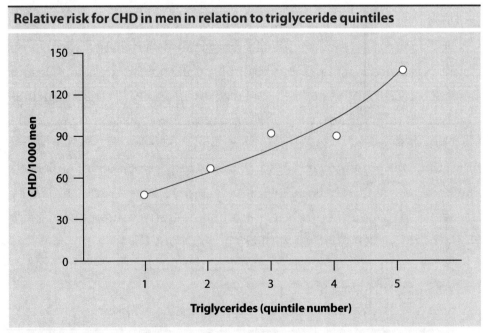

Figure 1.8 Relative risk for CHD in relation to quintiles of plasma fasting triglyceride levels. Triglyceride values vary with age. The quintile values are age adjusted. The border value at age 40–50 years between quintiles 1 and 2 and between 4 and 5 were 1.0 and 2.1 mmol/L, respectively. CHD, coronary heart disease. Adapted with permission from Carlson LA et al. Acta Med Scand 1985;218:207–211.

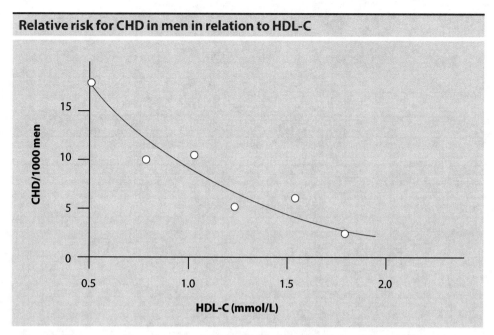

Figure 1.9 Relative risk for CHD in men in relation to concentration of HDL-C. Data from the Framingham study. CHD, coronary heart disease; HDL-C, high-density lipoprotein cholesterol. Reproduced from Gordon T et al. Am J Med 1977;62:704–714, ©1977, with permission from Excerpta Medica, Inc.

Chapter 2

From cholesterol to lipoproteins and apolipoproteins

Atherosclerosis

Since 1816, the year when the French chemist Chevreul discovered cholesterol, there has been an increasing interest in the role of cholesterol, and subsequently in the dyslipidaemias, as causal risk factors for atherosclerosis and its sequel clinical atherosclerosis. The role of blood lipids and lipid parameters as risk factors for clinical atherosclerosis started to become evident when methods to determine blood cholesterol became available at the beginning of the 20th century. These used the Liebermann–Burchard colour reaction, which is specific for cholesterol. Soon case–control studies were published showing that high plasma cholesterol levels were frequent in patients with CHD. It was soon discovered that cholesterol was not present in plasma as such but occurred in combination with proteins and other lipids in large molecules that circulate in the blood as particles called lipoproteins.

Lipoprotein particles

The lipoproteins are large particles composed of a protein shell containing a lipid core. The shell is made up of a specific class of proteins, the apolipoproteins (see below) and hydrophilic lipids, i.e. phospholipids and unesterified (free) cholesterol. The core contains the hydrophobic lipids (cholesterol esters and triglycerides). Each lipoprotein particle can contain many hundreds of cholesterol molecules. A schematic representation of the structure of a lipoprotein particle is shown in Figure 2.1.

Lipoprotein model

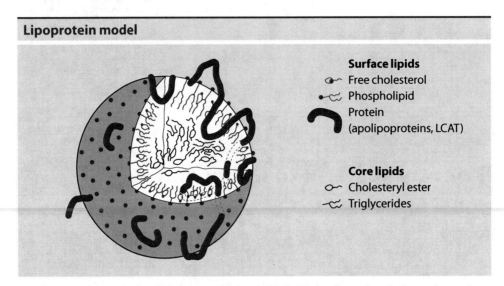

Surface lipids
- Free cholesterol
- Phospholipid
- Protein (apolipoproteins, LCAT)

Core lipids
- Cholesteryl ester
- Triglycerides

Figure 2.1 Lipoprotein model. The most hydrophobic lipids (triglycerides, cholesteryl esters) form a central droplet-like core, which is surrounded by more polar lipids (phospholipids, free cholesterol) at the water interface. Apolipoproteins are anchored by their more hydrophobic regions, with their more polar regions often exposed at the surface. LCAT, lecithin:cholesterol acyltransferase. Reproduced with permission from Durrington PN. Hyperlipidaemia: Diagnosis and Management. 2nd edition. London: Butterworth-Heinemann; 1995.

By means of advanced physico-chemical methods, it was shown that the plasma lipoproteins existed in different, well-defined classes. Using analytical and preparative ultracentrifugation, three major classes have been defined in fasting plasma:

- endogenous very low-density lipoproteins (VLDL),
- low-density lipoproteins (LDL), and
- high-density lipoproteins (HDL).

In non-fasting plasma there are also triglyceride-rich exogenous chylomicrons which carry alimentary fats (triglycerides and fat-soluble substances, e.g. certain vitamins).

Endogenous lipoprotein particles

The endogenous lipoprotein particles are synthesised in the liver and in the gut.

Very low-density lipoproteins

These are the major carrier of triglycerides and normally account for 10% of plasma cholesterol. In clinical practice, VLDL levels are not measured: the plasma triglyceride value is used as a measure of their concentration.

VLDL particles are secreted from the liver into the blood, where they transport triglycerides to peripheral tissues to be used as a source of energy or to be stored as fuel. VLDL undergoes extensive catabolism in the circulation, in particular losing triglycerides by the action of lipoprotein lipase. The fatty acids generated by this process are taken up by tissues, oxidised or stored in triglyceride droplets, and are eventually transformed into LDL particles, as shown in Figures 2.2 and 2.3.

It is worth noting that each VLDL particle has only one molecule of apoB which remains on the particle when it is being transformed into an LDL particle.

Low-density lipoproteins

These are the major carrier of plasma cholesterol and account for more than 50% of plasma cholesterol. Each LDL particle has one molecule of apoB (apoB100). They are generated in plasma from metabolised VLDL particles, always maintaining their apoB molecule as mentioned above. LDL is taken up by the liver and peripheral tissues, including the arterial

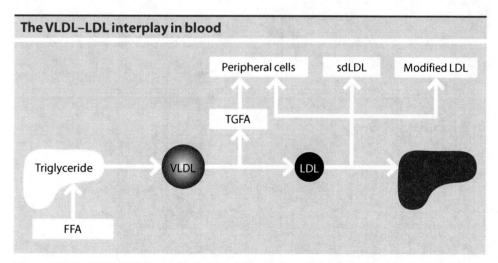

Figure 2.2 The VLDL–LDL interplay in blood. The triglyceride-rich very-low-density lipoprotein (VLDL) particle is synthesised in the liver with one molecule of apolipoprotein B (apoB) on the surface and triglycerides and cholesteryl esters in the core. The ripe particle is secreted into plasma where it undergoes delipidation by action of lipases. By this mechanism, VLDL successively loses triglyceride fatty acids (TGFA) from the core, which are taken up by peripheral cells. Eventually the lipoprotein particle, which retains its apoB molecule on the surface and its cholesteryl esters in the core, is turned into a cholesterol-rich low-density lipaoprotein (LDL) particle. LDL may then be taken up by hepatocytes or peripheral tissues, including arteries, through the action of the LDL receptor. LDL may also be metabolised to small dense LDL (sdLDL) by hepatic lipase or modified (oxidation, glycosylation). Plasma free fatty acids (FFA) derived from lipolysis in adipose tissue are important substrates for VLDL triglycerides.

wall, through the action of the LDL receptor, for which the single molecule of apoB on the particle surface is the ligand. Once inside cells, LDL delivers cholesterol after enzymatic digestion of the particle. Cholesterol cannot be broken down in the cells and therefore accumulates, particularly in foam cells – the hallmark of atherosclerosis. Cholesterol can, however, be removed from cells by the process of reverse cholesterol transport, as described below.

The VLDL–LDL interplay in blood

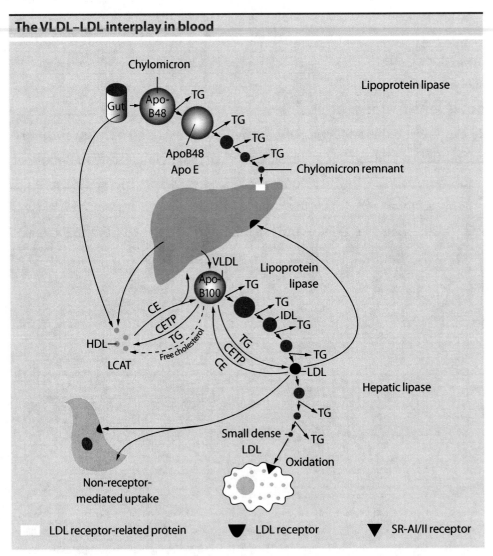

Figure 2.3 Metabolism of chylomicrons, VLDL, IDL and LDL. An outline of the major metabolic pathways by which chylomicron remnants and LDL are formed from chylomicrons and VLDL, respectively, and subsequently catabolised. HDL is secreted by the gut and liver and receives additional components during the metabolism of triglyceride-rich lipoproteins. Apo, apolipoprotein; CE, cholesteryl ester; CETP, cholesteryl ester transfer protein; HDL, high-density lipoprotein; IDL, intermediate-density lipoprotein; LCAT, lecithin:cholesterol acyltransferase; LDL, low-density lipoprotein; SR, scavenger receptor; TG, triglyceride; VLDL, very-low-density lipoprotein. Adapted with permission from Durrington PN. Hyperlipidaemia: Diagnosis and Management, 2nd Edition. London: Butterworth-Heinemann; 1995.

Small, dense LDL (sdLDL)

These are particles generated in plasma from mature LDL particles by the action of two enzymes, cholesteryl ester transfer protein (CETP) and hepatic lipase (HL). The first step in the transformation of LDL is that CETP exchanges one cholesterol molecule in LDL with a triglyceride molecule from VLDL. This is followed by lipolysis of the triglyceride by HL. The overall result is that LDL becomes smaller and denser. The resultant sdLDL particles are more easily oxidised and more atherogenic than the original LDL particle.

High-density lipoproteins

These are the smallest lipoprotein particles and carry only about 25% of total plasma cholesterol. The main apolipoproteins in HDL are apoA-I and apoA-II, which are synthesised in the liver and the gut. An important role of HDL in plasma lipid transport is its function in reverse cholesterol transport, the process by which cholesterol is picked up by HDL from peripheral tissues and via various intravascular processes is transported to the liver for excretion from the body.

Lipoprotein (a)

This is a unique lipoprotein consisting of an LDL particle linked to an apoA moiety. Apolipoprotein (a) is very similar to plasminogen in its structure and may inhibit fibrinolysis. As yet, clinical interest in Lp(a) is fairly weak, and for now Lp(a) can be measured only in a few laboratories.

Physiological transport functions of the endogenous lipoproteins

The major function of the endogenous plasma lipoproteins is to transport lipids between organs and tissues:

- VLDL transports triglyceride fatty acids from the liver to peripheral tissues for energy purposes.
- LDL transports cholesterol from the liver via VLDL to peripheral tissues for synthesis of cellular membranes and steroid hormones.
- HDL transports cholesterol from peripheral tissues to the liver for elimination from the body in bile.

Physiological transport functions of the exogenous lipoprotein particles

Chylomicrons are the largest lipoprotein particles – 'fat droplets' that are formed in the intestines and carry alimentary fat from the intestines through the thoracic lymph ducts into the blood. These triglyceride-rich particles each contain one molecule of apoB48 and small amounts of other lipoproteins (apoC, apoE) and cholesterol and phospholipids. Chylomicron triglycerides are hydrolysed in capillary beds by the action of lipoprotein lipase.

Most lipoprotein lipase is present in adipose tissue capillaries therefore most alimentary fatty acids released from chylomicrons enter adipose tissue for storage. Small amounts of the fatty acids are bound to albumin and transported to skeletal and myocardial muscles for oxidation to generate energy or to be stored as intracellular fat droplets which constitute energy stores. The redundant surface material of the shrinking chylomicron particle (apolipoproteins, free cholesterol, phospholipids) is taken up by the HDL pool. The remaining skeleton of the chylomicron particle –the chylomicron remnant – is circulated in the blood and eventually taken up by the liver (Figure 2.3).

Apolipoproteins

Apolipoproteins are the class of proteins that are present in lipoprotein particles. A large number have been have been identified and isolated (apoA, apoB, apoC, apoE and others). Their structure and function in lipid metabolism have been elucidated. They stabilise the shells of lipoprotein particles, give the particles their hydrophilic properties and have several effects in lipoprotein metabolism, such as acting as ligands for lipoprotein receptors and activation of lipid metabolism enzymes.

The major functions and effects of some of the apolipoproteins in lipoprotein metabolism are:

- The large apoB molecule, consisting of about 2500 amino acids, acts as a ligand of LDL for the LDL receptor. Mutations of apoB lead to diminished uptake of LDL from the blood, which causes familial hypercholesterolaemia (FH).

- Apolipoprotein A-I, containing approximately 250 amino acids is the major apolipoprotein of HDL. It is the key physiological activator of the plasma enzyme lecithin:cholesterol acyltransferase (LCAT). In addition, apoA-I is an acceptor of cell membrane cholesterol in reverse cholesterol transport.
- Apolipoprotein A-II is the second most important apolipoprotein in HDL.
- Apolipoprotein E is a component of chylomicron remnants and LDL and serves as a ligand for the LDL receptor and also for the LDL receptor-related protein. Apolipoprotein E exists in several isoforms, and homozygosity for one of these (apoE2) causes the severe but rare type III hyperlipidaemia.
- Apolipoprotein C-II is an activator of lipoprotein lipase. Lack of apoC-II leads to massive hypertriglyceridaemia.

  In routine clinical settings, apoB and apoA-I are the only apolipoprotein that are measured. They are used as indicators of concentrations of LDL/VLDL and HDL, respectively.

Chapter 3

Lipid testing

The main purposes of lipid testing are:
- Diagnosis and characterisation of dyslipidaemia, primary as well as secondary.
- Determination of lipid risk factors.
- Evaluation of lipid treatment.

Diagnosis

Diagnosis of dyslipidaemia, defined as an abnormal level of one or more of the plasma lipoproteins, requires the determination of the lipid profile. The standard lipid profile is sufficient for this aim and allows the detection of the presence of the Fredrickson types of hyperlipidaemia, although some special tests are required for the exact diagnosis of types I, III and V. The standard lipid profile will also detect and diagnose other dyslipidaemias, such as low levels of HDL-C and LDL-C (hypo- and abetalipoproteinaemia). However, the diagnosis of rare types of dyslipidaemia, such as LCAT deficiency and fish-eye disease, requires more elaborate tests.

Quantitative aspects

Diagnosis of the various dyslipidaemias requires that abnormal lipid and lipoprotein concentrations are defined and hence 'normal' values are specified. This is not easy for lipid values because they are strongly influenced by genetic, environmental and lifestyle factors. For example, in the USA and in many northern European countries, the statistical average for cholesterol is over 5.2 mmol/L (200 mg/dL); in contrast, the average is approximately 4 mmol/L (150 mg/dL) in many Asian countries. Historically, in the earlier part of the twentieth century, normal values were often established dogmatically. Thus, the normal cholesterol value was defined as ≤7.8 mmol/L (300 mg/dL): values below this were accepted as normal, and values above it were deemed to represent hypercholesterolaemia.

In order to overcome the problem of defining normal values for plasma lipids, 'target' values for the different lipid fractions have been tailored to accommodate the treatment requirements of different risk categories in the ATP III (Third Report of the Expert Panel on Detection, Evaluation, and Treatment of High Blood Cholesterol in Adults) of the US NCEP (US National Cholesterol Education Program). The relationship between plasma levels of the various lipids and the risk for clinical atherosclerosis is continuous, and therefore ATP III does not define a threshold values for use in risk prediction. Instead, ATP III classifies LDL-C, HDL-C and total-C into risk categories such as optimal, near or above optimal, borderline high, high and very high. Values so defined by ATP III for total-C, LDL-C and HDL-C are shown in Figure 3.1. In accordance with this classification, one might be inclined to set the old-fashioned normal level for total-C at 5.2 mmol/L (200 mg/dL), however use of the ATP III classification of cholesterol values is more attractive.

ATP III Classification of risk categories for LDL, total and HDL cholesterol			
	mmol/L	mg/dL	Category
LDL cholesterol	<2.6	<100	Optimal
	2.6–3.3	100–129	Near or above optimal
	3.4–4.1	130–159	Borderline high
	4.1–4.9	160–189	High
	≥4.9	≥190	Very high
Total cholesterol	<5.2	<200	Desirable
	5.2–6.2	200–239	Borderline high
	>6.2	≥240	High
HDL-cholesterol	<1.0	<40	Low
	≥1.6	≥60	High

Figure 3.1 ATP III Classification of risk categories for LDL, total and HDL cholesterol. ATP III, Third report of the Expert Panel on Detection, Evaluation, and Treatment of High Blood Cholesterol in Adults. HDL, high-density lipoprotein; LDL, low-density lipoprotein. Adapted from [11].

ATP III has classified values for plasma triglycerides into four categories in a similar way: normal, borderline high, high and very high, as shown in Figure 3.2.

Ground-breaking studies

Two important ground-breaking studies of lipid testing in the assessment of risk of clinical atherosclerosis appeared in the middle of the twentieth century: work by Fredrickson and co-workers at the National Institutes of Health (NIH) in Bethesda, USA, and data from the Framingham Heart Study.

Fredrickson and co-workers expanded lipid testing so that it no longer included only determination of cholesterol and triglyceride levels but also involved assessment of lipoproteins. They produced the first classification system for dyslipidaemias, later revised by a consensus group of the World Health Organization (WHO). The Fredrickson/WHO classification comprised six well-defined types of hyperlipidaemia, types I, IIa, IIb, III, IV and V [8]. A summary of this ground-breaking system is given in Figure 3.3. Of note is that this system is only useful for hyperlipidaemias and not for dyslipidaemias in general because it does not include, for example, abnormalities of HDL.

The Fredrickson/WHO classification is based on a combination of determination of cholesterol and triglyceride levels and the analysis of lipoproteins by qualitative lipoprotein electrophoresis. Although lipoprotein electrophoresis is rarely used nowadays, the terminology of the Fredrickson classification system is still used as a short-hand notation for lipoprotein disorders, which are now and assessed using

ATP III classification of risk categories for triglycerides		
mmol/L	mg/dL	Category
<1.7	<150	Normal
1.7–2.2	150–199	Borderline high
2.2–5.5	200–499	High
>5.5	>500	Very high

Figure 3.2 ATP III classification of risk categories for triglycerides. ATP III, Third report of the Expert Panel on Detection, Evaluation, and Treatment of High Blood Cholesterol in Adults. Adapted from [11].

more accurate, quantitative methods. This opened the door to the recognition and use of LDL as the key important plasma lipid risk factor for clinical atherosclerosis.

The second ground breaking study, at least equally important in the progress of the evaluation of risk factors for clinical atherosclerosis, was the shift from case–control studies to the prospective reports on risk factors for clinical atherosclerosis emanating from Framingham, USA [5]. The basic concept of the Framingham Heart Study was that a causative risk factor must be present before the disease arrives on the clinical horizon. The Framingham Heart Study is still ongoing, now publishing results from the offspring of Framingham participants; the Framingham Offspring Study is discussed further in Chapter 6.

Guidelines for lipid testing and lipid management

Many guidelines for lipid testing and lipid management, as well as for prevention of CVD, have appeared during the last two decades. Two major guidelines are of special interest for this review, one emanating from the USA [9] and the other from Europe [10].

The American guideline, ATP III from the NCEP, has become the international foundation for guidelines. The US National Heart, Lung and Blood Institute has issued several ATP guidelines since the end of the twentieth century (ATP I, ATP II and ATP III). ATP III constitutes

Fredrickson/WHO classification of types of hyperlipidaemia		
Type	**Lipoprotein increased**	**Lipid increased**
I	Chylomicrons	Triglycerides* and cholesterol
IIA	LDL	Cholesterol
IIB	LDL	Cholesterol and triglycerides
	VLDL	Cholesterol and triglycerides
III	Beta–VLDL	Cholesterol*
	IDL Chylomicron remnants	Triglycerides*
IV	VLDL	Triglycerides
V	Chylomicron	Triglycerides* and cholesterol
	VLDL	Triglycerides* and cholesterol

Figure 3.3 Fredrickson/WHO classification of types of hyperlipidaemia. *Massive elevation. IDL, intermediate-density lipoprotein; LDL, low-density lipoprotein; VLDL, very low-density lipoprotein; WHO, World Health Organization.

the NCEP's updated clinical guidelines for cholesterol testing and management. An executive summary of ATP III was published in 2001 [11], followed by an ATP III Update in 2004 [12].

The European guideline was first published in 1994. The present updated guideline is the Fourth Joint Task Force of the European Society of Cardiology and other societies on cardiovascular prevention in clinical practice, published in 2007 [10].

Chapter 4

Lipid profiles

The lipid profile evaluates a person´s blood lipid status quantitatively. It came into use when, in addition to cholesterol and triglycerides, methods to determine LDL-C and HDL-C became available in routine clinical practice. Subsequently, attempts to advance the evaluation of risk for clinical atherosclerosis have continued, in order to improve prevention and treatment of the disease. In this respect, as described later in this chapter, two major new lipid risk factors are beginning to be used in everyday clinical work:

- non-HDL-C and
- apolipoproteins.

There are three types of lipid profile currently in use in the daily clinical setting:

- classical standard lipid profile,
- cholesterol-based lipid profile and
- apolipoprotein-based lipid profile.

The classical standard lipid profile

The classical standard lipid profile shown in Figure 4.1 has been used for many years in routine clinical practice. It continues to be used in many clinical locations and in studies on the effect of lipid-modulating drugs. It provides the physician a reasonable level of basic information about a patient´s lipid risk factor status.

The lipid profile is determined after fasting overnight (10–12 hours). During treatment of lipid disorders, the profile is checked regularly to evaluate the lipid response to the treatment. Once lipid goals have been

Classic standard lipid profile
• Total cholesterol
• Triglycerides
• LDL-cholesterol
• HDL-cholesterol

Figure 4.1 Classic standard lipid profile. HDL, High-density lipoprotein; LDL, low-density lipoprotein.

reached and the treatment is maintaining a stable state, the lipid profile is checked every 6–12 months. For example, a general recommendation is that the lipid profile should be checked every year in adults with diabetes.

A limitation of the classical standard lipid profile as determined in most clinical laboratories today is that LDL-C is not estimated directly but instead is estimated indirectly by calculation according to the Friedewald equation. Friedewald equation for estimation of LDL-C (TG, triglyceride):

Values in mmol/L: LDL-C = total-C - HDL-C - TG/2.2

Values in mg/dL: LDL-C = total-C - HDL-C - TG/5

In this equation, TG/2.2 and TG/5, respectively, provides a very rough estimate of VLDL-C, which can vary substantially from day to day in a given patient. Furthermore, the formula can only be used for triglyceride values below 4.5 mmol/L (400 mg/dL).

When LDL-C is calculated in this way, it contains contributions from intermediate-density lipoprotein cholesterol (IDL-C) and Lp(a)-C. An aspect to bear in mind is that the result is obtained from three different measurements, each of which is subject to methodological error. Furthermore, the calculation is based upon the assumption that the fasting triglyceride value multiplied by a constant can give an exact value for VLDL-C.

It is expected, however, that in the near future, most laboratories will estimate LDL-C by direct, LDL-C-specific methods

Cholesterol-based lipid profiles and non-HDL-C

In striving to obtain as good a prediction as possible for the risk for clinical atherosclerosis, the classical standard lipid profile has been expanded.

Figure 4.2 lists the measures which are included in the current expanded cholesterol-based lipid profile. Criteria for obtaining the expanded profile are the same as for the classical standard profile.

The major difference between the expanded profile and the classical standard profile is the addition of non-HDL-C as a measure. Non-HDL-C is obtained by subtracting HDL-C from total-C. It is composed of LDL-C plus VLDL-C, plus the tiny amounts of cholesterol carried by Lp(a), i.e. it is is the sum of all cholesterol in apoB-containing lipoproteins.

Non-HDL-C has been advocated by the NCEP ATP III as an indicator of total-C in the atherogenic lipoproteins VLDL and LDL. As would be expected, it is highly correlated with the concentration of apoB and therefore can be regarded as a good indicator of the amount of apoB-containing lipoprotein.

The two ratios total-C/HDL-C and LDL-C/HDL-C are easily calculated from the values obtained in both the standard and expanded lipid profiles. Their utility is based on the assumption that they should give an estimate of the balance between cholesterol influx (LDL) and outflux (HDL) to and from the atherosclerotic plaque, as depicted in Figure 4.3.

Apolipoprotein-based lipid profiles

Although the apolipoproteins are proteins, the profile based on them is nevertheless called a lipid profile because apolipoproteins are measures of

Classic standard lipid profile

- Total cholesterol
- Triglycerides
- LDL-cholesterol
- HDL-cholesterol
- Ratio total cholesterol/HDL-cholesterol
- Non-HDL-cholesterol

Options:

- Ratio LDL-cholesterol/HDL-cholesterol
- Lipoprotein (a)

LDL-cholesterol is calculated by the Friedewald formula (see above)

Figure 4.2 Cholesterol-based lipid profile. HDL, High-density lipoprotein; LDL, low-density lipoprotein.

lipoprotein. The apolipoprotein-based lipid profile has three components, listed in Figure 4.4. One of its advantages is that because triglycerides are not included it can be taken in the non-fasting state, i.e. during the day and without disrupting ordinary life.

Apolipoprotein B provides an estimate of the number of circulating atherogenic lipoprotein particles containing apoB (VLDL, IDL, LDL and Lp[a]), because each of these particles contains one and only one molecule of the large apoB molecule. Apolipoprotein A-I, which is the major apolipoprotein of HDL, gives an approximate measure of the amount of circulating protective HDL. Of note with respect to apoA-I is that the subfractions of HDL, such as HDL_2 and HDL_3, contain different amounts of apoA-I per particle. Also, the ratio apoB/apoA-I is believed to give an idea of the balance between in- and outflux of cholesterol to/from the arteries (Figure 4.3).

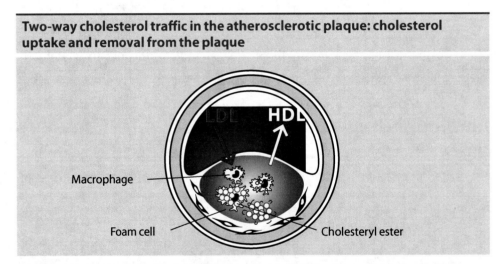

Two-way cholesterol traffic in the atherosclerotic plaque: cholesterol uptake and removal from the plaque

Macrophage

Foam cell

Cholesteryl ester

Figure 4.3 Two-way cholesterol traffic in the atherosclerotic plaque: cholesterol uptake and removal from the plaque. Cholesterol is derived from the uptake of modified LDL into macrophages and stored as droplets of cholesteryl ester, which turns the macrophage into a foam cell. After cell death the droplets accumulate in the extracellular space, cholesterol is removed by HDL and transported to the liver for excretion. HDL-C, high-density lipoprotein cholesterol; LDL-C, low-density lipoprotein cholesterol.

Apolipoprotein-based lipid profile

- apoB
- apoA-I
- Ratio apoB/apoA-I

Figure 4.4 Apolipoprotein-based lipid profile.

The AMORIS study

At the end of the 1990s several papers began to appear suggesting that apolipoproteins, particularly apoB and apoA, might be of value as risk factors in the prediction of atherosclerosis risk. But this idea did not immediately gain a hearing. However, a breakthrough for the use of apoB and apoA-I as risk factors came with the large AMORIS (Apolipoprotein Mortality Risk) study published in *The Lancet* in 2001 [13]. The AMORIS study was a prospective study. The participants were referred mainly from health check-ups. This original AMORIS study was sampled in 1985–1989 and comprised about 175,000 men and women in Stockholm, of whom nearly 1200 (864 men) suffered from a fatal myocardial infarction during the 5½ years of follow up. The mean ages for men and women were 47.1 and 49.7 years, respectively.

The main results of the original AMORIS study are shown in Figure 4.5. The relative risk for the three top quartiles versus those in the bottom quartile were calculated for all variables and are presented as the risk ratios in this figure. As shown in Figure 4.5, in both sexes there was a strong increase in risk with increasing levels of triglycerides, apoB, LDL cholesterol and the apoB/apoA-I ratio, but the relationship for total-C was weaker, particularly for women. Numerically the steepest increase in risk for myocardial infarction was obtained for the apoB/apoA-I ratio: in men, the risk increased about 3.8-fold for those in the top quartiles compared with those in the lowest. On the other hand, there was a strong negative relation between both HDL-C and apoA-I and the risk of myocardial infarction, i.e. higher levels correlated with a protective effect. AMORIS did not, however, measure baseline HDL-C, blood pressure, smoking, body mass index or diabetes

Advanced lipid testing

Advanced lipid testing is a concept that applies to the evaluation of lipid risk factors beyond standard lipid profiles. One typical aspect of advanced lipid testing is the determination of subfractions to the three major lipoprotein classes, VLDL, LDL and HDL, believed to be more or less atherogenic (VLDL, LDL) or protective (HDL). Another is determination of the number of lipoprotein particles in a given (sub)class of lipoproteins. The

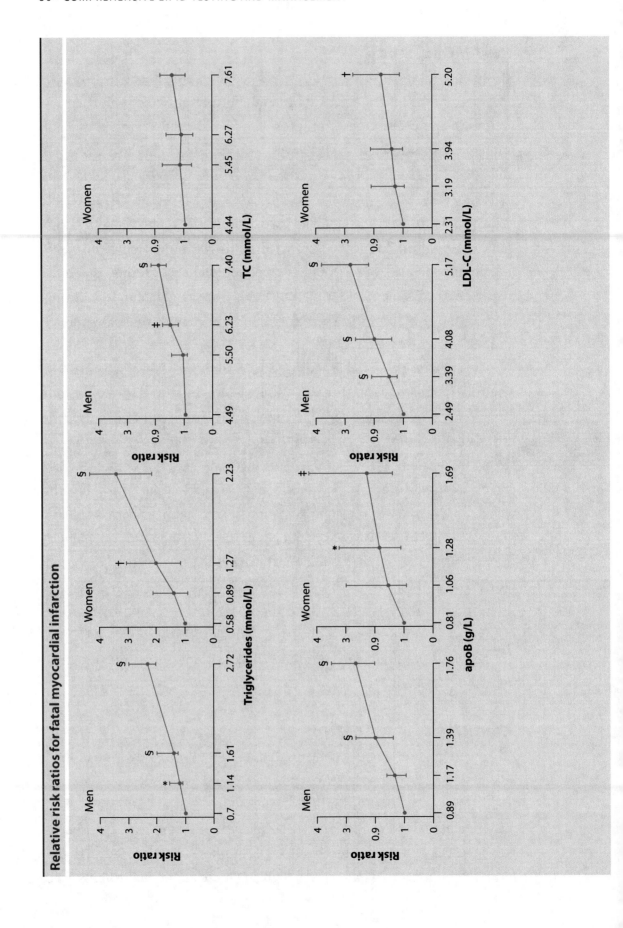

Relative risk ratios for fatal myocardial infarction

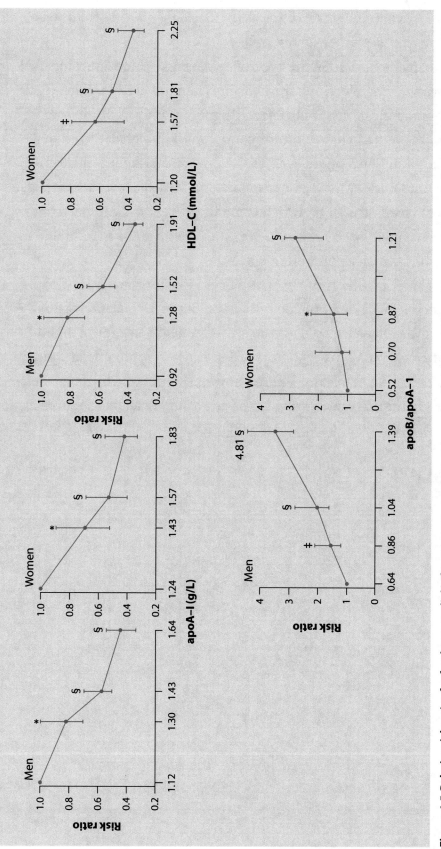

Figure 4.5 Relative risk ratios for fatal myocardial infarction, adjusted for fasting and log transformed for age for men and women in the original AMORIS study. Values are for people with triglycerides <4.5 mmol/L by quartiles (mean values shown). Vertical bars=95% CIs. *p <0.05; †p <0.01; ‡p <0.001; §p <0.0001. apo, apolipoprotein; C, cholesterol; HDL-C, high-density lipoprotein cholesterol; LDL-C, low-density lipoprotein cholesterol; T, total cholesterol. Reproduced with permission from Walldius G et al. Lancet 2001;358:2026–2033.

content of an advanced lipid testing battery may depend on the purpose of the testing – clinical or basic research.

Advanced methods used in this type of lipid testing are two variantsof electrophoresis (zone electrophoresis or gradient gel electrophoresis), four different applications of ultracentrifugation (analytical ultracentrifugation, sequential flotation ultracentrifugation, density gradient ultracentrifugation and single vertical spin density gradient ultracentrifugation) and nuclear magnetic resonance (NMR) spectroscopy. The most advanced method is NMR, which in minutes gives an NMR spectrum that is deconvoluted by computer; the results are given as the number of particles in the major lipoprotein classes.

One of the clinically most useful pieces of information that the advanced technologies can provide is the level of the highly atherogenic sdLDL. However, advanced lipid testing is usually available only in highly specialised clinical chemistry laboratories and a few advanced lipid research laboratories. Thus, in general, advanced lipid testing does not have a place in routine lipid testing in the clinic but instead is a tool for advanced research in clinical lipidology.

Chapter 5

Lipid testing and prediction of coronary heart disease

Prediction of CHD risk based on risk factor estimation was first used by the Framingham study in the early 1970s. The variables were age, sex, cholesterol, blood pressure, smoking and diabetes [14]. Risk prediction based on Framingham data was improved in the 1980s by addition of the 'negative' lipid risk factor HDL-C [15]. Subsequently, there have been further developments in risk prediction. These and the present status of risk prediction in clinical atherosclerosis have recently been reviewed by Wilson [16], including an overview of the major different risk prediction algorithms (Figure 5.1).

The two comprehensive guidelines ATP III [11] and euroSCORE [10] have recently published risk factor algorithms for prediction of CHD. From the early days, risk predictions have focused on single risk factors such as blood lipids or hypertension, however the focus has been changed to a multifactorial view of risk assessment in these guidelines.

An example of the effect of multiple risk factors on the risk of fatal CVD as predicted by the ratio total-C/HDL-C is given in Figure 5.2, The tremendous impact of both smoking and systolic blood pressure is striking and illustrates the usefulness of the multifactorial approach in forecasting risk.

Factors predicting the highest risk

According to ATP III, the highest risk of death or a serious cardiovascular event resulting from CHD is conferred by the presence of CHD itself, along with other manifestations of clinical atherosclerosis. The highest risk of a CHD event within 10 years is defined as 20% per 10 years, i.e. 20 persons out of 100 with the presence of CHD (myocardial infarction, angina pectoris) or other manifestations of clinical atherosclerosis (Figure 1.1) are expected to suffer from a new CHD event.

In prediction of serious cardiovascular events, risk equivalents to the presence of CHD are:

- manifestations of clinical atherosclerosis,
- diabetes and
- the presence of sufficient multiple risk factors to predict that the 10-year risk for CHD is >20%.

Further prediction of 10-year risk

The risk factors used by ATP III to determine LDL-C goals for treatment are shown in Figure 5.3, along with the criteria used to ascertain to presence of each factor.

Examples of CHD event prediction with risk factor algorithms				
	Wilson et al. 1998 [17]	ATP III 2001 [11]	Assmann et al. 2002 [18]	euroSCORE 2003 [19]
Data source	Framingham	Framingham	PROCAM	Europe
Age interval (years)	5 years	5 years	5 years	5 years
Sex	M, F	M, F	M	M, F
BP levels	JNC-VI	Systolic BP	Systolic BP	Systolic BP
BP therapy	No	Yes	No	No
Cholesterol	Yes	Yes	No	Yes
HDL cholesterol	Yes	Yes	Yes	No*
LDL cholesterol	Optional	No	Yes	No
Cigarettes	Yes	Yes	Yes	Yes
Diabetes mellitus	Yes	No	Yes	Yes
Baseline heart disease	ECG-LVH	No	MI history	No
CHD event	Total CHD	Hard CHD	Next Hard CHD	CHD death

Figure 5.1 Examples of CHD event prediction with risk factor algorithms. ATP III, Third report of the Expert Panel on Detection, Evaluation, and Treatment of High Blood Cholesterol in Adults; BP, blood pressure; CHD, coronary heart disease; ECG, electrocardiography; euroSCORE, European System for Cardiac Operative Risk Evaluation; F, female; JNC, Joint National Committee; LVH, left ventricular hypertrophy; M, male; PROCAM, Prospective Cardiovascular Münster investigation. *Total-C/HDL-C ratio given. Adapted from [16].

There are two steps for the assessment of cardiovascular risk for people who are not in the highest risk category. First, the number of risk factors is counted (Figure 5.4). For people with multiple risk factors (2+) the risk is then calculated from the Framingham risk score for men and women (Figure 5.4).

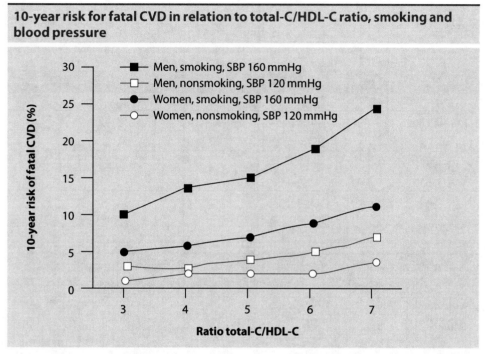

10-year risk for fatal CVD in relation to total-C/HDL-C ratio, smoking and blood pressure

Figure 5.2 10-year risk for fatal CVD in relation to total-C/HDL-C ratio, smoking and blood pressure. Data are for men and women aged 60 years with and without risk factors, based on a risk function derived from the SCORE project. C, cholesterol; CVD, cardiovascular disease; HDL, high-density lipoprotein; SBP, systolic blood pressure; TC, total cholesterol. Data from [11].

ATP III major risk factors that modify LDL goals*

Risk factor	Criteria for presence of risk factor
Cigarette smoking	Current smoking
Hypertension	BP ≥140/90mmHg or on antihypertensive medication
Low HDL cholesterol	<40 mg/dL†
Family history of premature CHD	CHD in male first-degree relative <55 years
	CHD in female first-degree relative <65 years
Age	Men ≥45 years;
	Women ≥55 years

Figure 5.3 ATP III major risk factors (exclusive of LDL cholesterol) that modify LDL goals. *Diabetes is regarded as a CHD risk equivalent. †HDL cholesterol ≥60 mg/dL counts as a "negative" risk factor and its presence removes 1 risk factor from the total count. ATP III, Third report of the Expert Panel on Detection, Evaluation, and Treatment of High Blood Cholesterol in Adults; CHD, coronary heart disease; HDL, high-density lipoprotein; LDL, low-density lipoprotein. Adapted from [11].

Framingham risk scoring to estimate 10-year risk for developing CHD

MEN

Age (years)	Points		Age (years)	Points
20–34	–9		55–59	8
35–39	–4		60–64	10
40–44	0		65–69	11
45–49	3		70–74	12
50–54	6		75–79	13

Total cholesterol		Points				
mg/dL	mmol/L	Age 20–39 y	Age 40–49 y	Age 50–59 y	Age 60–69 y	Age 70–79 y
<160	4.1	0	0	0	0	0
160–199	4.1–5.2	4	3	2	1	0
200–239	5.2–6.2	7	5	3	1	0
240–279	6.2–7.2	9	6	4	2	1
≥280	<7.2	11	8	5	3	1

Smoking	Points				
	Age 20–39 y	Age 40–49 y	Age 50–59 y	Age 60–69 y	Age 70–79 y
Nonsmoker	0	0	0	0	0
Smoker	8	5	3	1	1

HDL, mg/dL	mmol/L	Points		Systolic BP, mmHg	If untreated	If treated
≥60	≥1.6	–1		<120	0	0
50–59	1.3–1.5	0		120–129	0	1
40–49	1.0–1.3	1		130–139	1	2
<40	<1.0	2		140–159	1	2
				≥160	2	3

Point total	10-year risk		Point total	10-year risk		Point total	10-year risk
<0	<1		6	2		13	12
0	1		7	3		14	16
1	1		8	4		15	20
2	1		9	5		16	25
3	1		10	6		≥17	≥30
4	1		11	8			
5	2		12	10			

Figure 5.4 Framingham risk scoring to estimate 10-year risk for developing CHD. BP, blood pressure; CHD, coronary heart disease; HDL, high-density lipoprotein; y, years. Adapted with permission from Adult Treatment Panel III. JAMA 2001;285:2486–2497.

Framingham risk scoring to estimate 10-year risk for developing CHD

WOMEN

Age (years)	Points		Age (years)	Points
20–34	–7		55–59	8
35–39	–3		60–64	10
40–44	0		65–69	12
45–49	3		70–74	14
50–54	6		75–79	16

Total cholesterol		Points				
mg/dL	mmol/L	Age 20–39 y	Age 40–49 y	Age 50–59 y	Age 60–69 y	Age 70–79 y
<160	4.1	0	0	0	0	0
160–199	4.1–5.2	4	3	2	1	1
200–239	5.2–6.2	8	6	4	2	1
240–279	6.2–7.2	11	8	5	3	2
≥280	<7.2	13	10	7	4	2

Smoking	Points				
	Age 20–39 y	Age 40–49 y	Age 50–59 y	Age 60–69 y	Age 70–79 y
Nonsmoker	0	0	0	0	0
Smoker	9	7	4	2	1

HDL, mg/dL	mmol/L	Points
≥60	≥1.6	–1
50–59	1.3–1.5	0
40–49	1.0–1.3	1
<40	<1.0	2

Systolic BP, mmHg	If untreated	If treated
<120	0	0
120–129	1	3
130–139	2	4
140–159	3	5
≥160	4	6

Point total	10-year risk	Point total	10-year risk	Point total	10-year risk
<9	<1	14	2	20	11
9	1	15	3	21	14
10	1	16	4	22	17
11	1	17	5	23	22
12	1	18	6	24	27
13	2	19	8	≥25	≥30

EuroSCORE

This has produced simple but instructive risk charts for asymptomatic people (no heart disease, no diabetes), giving the 10-year risk of fatal CVD on the basis of age, gender, smoking, systolic blood pressure and total-C (or the ratio of total-C/HDL-C). The charts are available for two European populations (Figures 5.5 and 5.6):

- Low-risk countries (Belgium, France, Greece, Italy Luxembourg, Spain, Switzerland and Portugal) and
- High-risk countries (all other European countries).

The charts are easy to use for rapid determination of a person's 10-year risk for a fatal cardiovascular event:

- Select high- or low-risk chart, as appropriate.
- Choose the columns for women or men.
- Opt for smoking or non-smoking status.
- Within the resulting block of data, identify the square that correlates with the cholesterol and blood pressure and read the risk value from it.

As an example, the risk for 65-year-old Italian female non-smoker who has a systolic blood pressure of 165 mmHg and cholesterol of 7.2 mmol/L is 4% (Figure 5.6); i.e. of 100 such women, four are predicted to suffer a fatal event during the coming 10 years. The 10-year risk for a 60-year-old British male smoker who has a systolic blood pressure of 180 mmHg and cholesterol of 5 mmol/L would be 21%. (Figure 5.5).

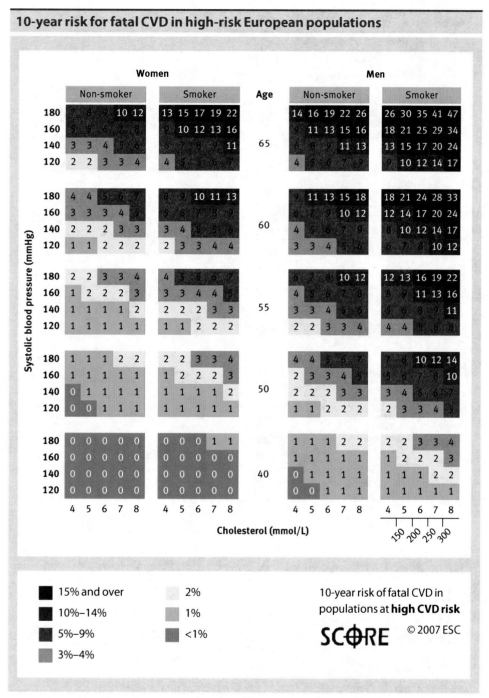

Figure 5.5 SCORE chart: 10-year risk for fatal CVD in European populations at high risk for CVD, based on age, gender, smoking, systolic blood pressure and total cholesterol. CVD, cardiovascular disease. Reproduced with permission from European guidelines on cardiovascular disease prevention in clinical practice: executive summary. Eur J Cardiovasc Prev and Rehab 2007;14(Suppl 2):E1–E40. © The European Society of Cardiology.

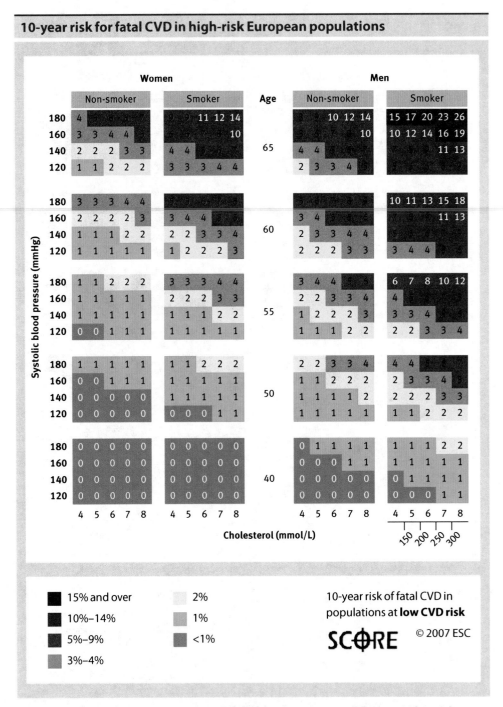

10-year risk for fatal CVD in high-risk European populations

Figure 5.6 SCORE chart: 10-year risk for fatal CVD in European populations at low risk for CVD based on age, gender, smoking, systolic blood pressure and total cholesterol. CVD, cardiovascular disease. Reproduced with permission from European guidelines on cardiovascular disease prevention in clinical practice: executive summary. Eur J Cardiovasc Prev and Rehab 2007;14(Suppl 2):E1–E40. © The European Society of Cardiology.

Chapter 6

Lipid risk factors in prediction of coronary heart disease – is any one factor best?

The fact that several components of dyslipidaemia have been shown to be significant risk factors for clinical atherosclerosis has raised the question of whether any single factor is outstanding in this regard. Such a factor would be the first-line choice in lipid testing to assess a patient´s risk for a heart attack or ischaemic stroke. Trying to answer this question, there have been four sufficiently large studies that have each made comparisons of the risk associated with different lipid factors within a single patient cohort: the Women´s Health Study [20], the Framingham Offspring Study [21], the AMORIS new (second) study [22] and the INTERHEART study [7].

The Women's Health Study

This comprised 15,632 healthy women with a mean age of 54 years, followed up for 10 years. Their mean body mass index was 26.3, 12% were smokers, 3% had diabetes and 25% had a history of hypertension. The endpoint was cardiovascular events after the start of the study (non-fatal myocardial infarction, non-fatal stroke, revascularisation procedures and cardiovascular-related death).

Subjects' median values for total-C, LDL-C, HDL-C and non-HDL-C were, respectively, 5.3 mmol/L (206 mg/dL), 3.2 (124), 1.27 (49) and 4.0 (155), and for apoB and apoA-I were 140 and 99 mg/dL. There was a strong correlation between non-HDL-C and apoB, $r=0.87$. Median values for the ratios total-C/HDL-C and apoB/apoA-I were 4.1 and 0.71, respectively.

A first-ever cardiovascular endpoint occurred in 464 of the participants. All of the measured lipid parameters were, after adjustment for age, blood pressure, body mass index, diabetes and current smoking, strongly associated with risk of future cardiovascular events ($p < 0.001$). The strongest association was for non-HDL-C and apoB, with hazard ratios (HR) for the highest quintile compared to the lowest of 2.51 and 2.50 (Figure 6.1), both being more strongly associated with the endpoint than either total-C or LDL-C. Of considerable importance was the strong association of high-sensitivity (hs) C-reactive protein (CRP) with the occurrence of new cardiovascular events.

Furthermore, the results suggested that the ratio total-C/HDL-C is superior to total-C or LDL-C in terms of predictive value, in contrast to euroSCORE which appears to favour the use of total-C in isolation.

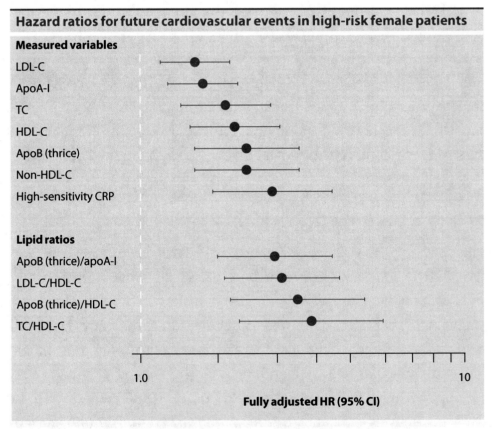

Figure 6.1 Hazard ratios for future cardiovascular events high-risk female patients in the extreme quintiles of each measured variable. HRs adjusted for age (years), blood pressure (Framingham categories), diabetes, current smoking status and body mass index. Apo, apolipoprotein; CI, confidence interval; CRP, C-reactive protein; HDL-C, high-density lipoprotein cholesterol; HR, hazard ratio; LDL-C, low-density lipoprotein cholesterol; TC, total cholesterol. Data from [20].

Conclusions

The author's conclusions were that non-HDL-C and the ratio total-C/HDL-C were as good as or better than apolipoprotein fractions in the prediction of future cardiovascular events. After adjustment for risk factors, hs-CRP added prognostic information beyond that conveyed by all lipid measures.

The Framingham Offspring Study

This followed 3322 apparently healthy individuals (53% females) with a mean age of 51 years for 15 years. CHD events were defined as myocardial infarction, angina pectoris, coronary insufficiency, or death due to CHD.

There were 291 first CHD events. In men, non-HDL-C, apoB, total-C/HDL-C and apoB/apoA-I were positively associated with a CHD risk of approximately the same magnitude and statistical significance, while total-C and LDL-C were not (limited statistical power). Apolipoprotein A-I and HDL-C were associated with a reduced risk of CHD.

In women, apoB, total-C/HDL-C and apoB/apoA-I and non-HDL-C were all associated with an increased risk, but total-C and LDL-C were not.

With more complex statistical analysis using the C-index and the receiver operating characteristic (ROC) curves for the ratios total-C/HDL-C and apoB/apoA-I, near equivalence of performance for these two ratios was demonstrated.

Conclusions

The authors' main conclusion was that the results indicate that the apoB/apoA-I ratio is the best single lipoprotein variable for quantification of coronary risk.

The second AMORIS study

This comprised 69,000 men and 57,000 women for whom there was no information on diagnosis or treatment at entry, with a mean age of 55 years and an average follow up of 8 years. The background for AMORIS was that cholesterol-related indices such as can be obtained with the apolipoprotein-based lipid profile described in Figure 4.4, are generally used to define the overall lipid-related risk of clinical atherosclerosis. However, recent work has suggested that apoB and apoA-I, and particularly their ratio (apoB/apoA-I), are more effective markers than plasma lipids in this regard. In the AMORIS study the purpose was to evaluate if the apoB/apoA-I ratio was superior to those of the cholesterol-based lipid profile in predicting the risk for fatal myocardial infarction.

The endpoint of the study was fatal myocardial infarction or sudden death, cases being obtained from the Swedish death register. Mean basal values for lipids were, in mmol/L (mg/dL), total-C 6.1 (235), triglycerides 1.6 (130), LDL-C 4.0 (155), HDL-C 1.4 (54), non-HDL-C 4.7 (180) and for both apoB and apoA-I 1.4 g/L, with a total-C/HDL-C ratio of 4.8 and an apoB/apoA-I ratio of 1.0. Average follow-up time was 8 years, during which time 1183 men and 560 women died from acute myocardial infarction.

For both sexes apoB was strongly and positively related ($p < 0.0001$) and apoA-I strongly and negatively related ($p < 0.0001$) to the risk of fatal myocardial infarction (Figure 6.2)

The risk functions for fatal myocardial infarction in relation to the two ratios apoB/apoA-I and total-C/HDL-C are shown in Figure 6.3. In both sexes there was a much steeper increase in risk for the apolipoprotein ratio than for the cholesterol ratio. Furthermore, when the apoB/apoA-I ratio was adjusted for age and each of the cholesterol ratios, the trend remained highly significant.

Conclusions

The authors' main conclusion was that the results indicate that the apoB/apoA-I ratio is the best single lipoprotein variable for quantification of coronary risk.

The INTERHEART study

This study is briefly described earlier (p. 3). The nine main global risk factors for myocardial infarction that emerged from it are listed in Figure 1.3. Among these the apoB/apoA-I ratio had the greatest power of risk prediction, with a PAR value of 49% compared with, for example, 18% for hypertension. Lipid analyses were carried out on samples taken in the non-fasting state, which does not affect values for total-C, HDL-C, apoB or apoA-I but precludes meaningful determination of triglycerides and thus invalidates the calculation of LDL-C using the Friedewald formula, hence LDL-C/HDL-C ratios were not reported in the INTERHEART study [7]. The mean concentrations of lipids and

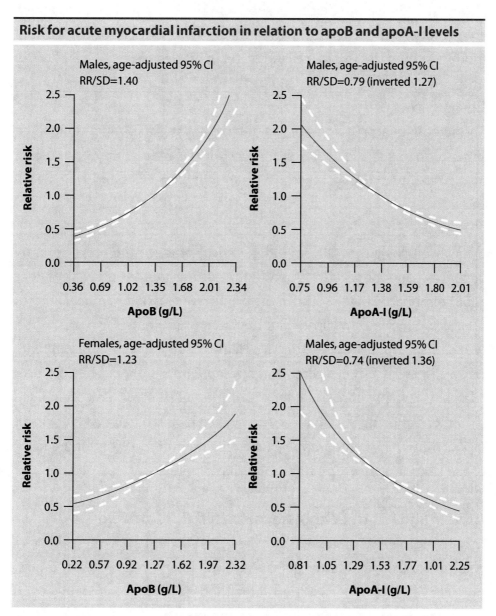

Figure 6.2 Age-adjusted relative risk for acute myocardial infarction, in relation to apoB and apoA-I levels in AMORIS study for males and females. RR/SD values and 95% CI levels are indicated (dashed lines). Relative risk (RR) values are expressed with one standard deviation (SD) as the unit change for each variable. Apo, apolipoprotein; CI, confidence interval. Reproduced with permission from Walldius G et al. Clin Chem Lab Med 2004;42:1355–1363.

lipid ratios were presented for all ethnic groups in that study but are not discussed here.

The risk of myocardial infarction is shown in Figure 6.4. Lipids and apolipoproteins are shown in the top panel and the total-C/HDL-C and apoB/apoA-I ratios are shown in the bottom panel. Apolipoprotein B and non-HDL-C were the strongest positive lipid risk predictors, apoA-I the strongest negative predictor. As shown in the bottom panel, the apoB/apoA-I ratio was associated with a much stronger risk for myocardial infarction than the total-C/HDL-C ratio in all deciles.

Conclusions

The authors' interpretation was that the non-fasting apoB/apoA-I ratio was superior to any of the cholesterol ratios for the estimation of the risk of myocardial infarction in all ethnic groups, in both sexes and at all ages.

Summary

It has been suggested that in daily clinical practice the more recently developed apolipoprotein-based lipid profile should replace the older cholesterol-based lipid profile in the prediction of risk for clinical athero-sclerosis. There are positive and negative arguments for both. In the two clinical studies – the Women's Health Study and the Framingham Offspring Study – the cholesterol- and apolipoprotein-based lipid profiles were equally good predictors of future cardiovascular events. On the other hand, in the two large epidemiological studies – AMORIS and INTERHEART – the apoB/apoA-I ratio was a significantly better predictor of the risk for myocardial infarction than the ratio total-C/HDL-C.

Advantages of the cholesterol-based lipid profile

In both the medical profession and the general population, there is a long tradition of using cholesterol has as a risk factor for myocardial infarction. For years it has been important in lifestyle health improvement and as a target for treatment by both diet and drugs.

The importance of 'bad' cholesterol (LDL) as well as 'good' cho-lesterol (HDL) is now well known not only to physicians but also to patients. Campaigns and guidelines have long been focused on the role of cholesterol in the development of and risk for clinical atherosclerosis, not least for the prevention and treatment of this disease. A shift from cholesterol to apolipoproteins for determination of risk and choice of treatment might cause considerable confusion not only for the medical profession but, as important, for the laymen as well. Last but not least,

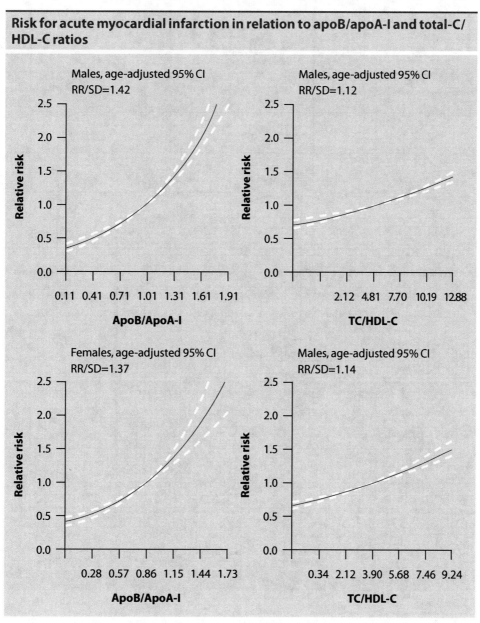

Figure 6.3 Age-adjusted relative risk for acute myocardial infarction, in relation to apoB/apoA-I and TC/HDL-C ratios in AMORIS study for males and females. RR/SD values and 95% CI levels are indicated (dotted lines). Relative risk (RR) values are expressed with one standard deviation (SD) as the unit change for each variable. Apo, apolipoprotein; CI, confidence interval; HDL-C, high-density lipoprotein cholesterol; TC, total cholesterol. Reproduced with permission from Walldius G et al. Clin Chem Lab Med 2004;42:1355–1363.

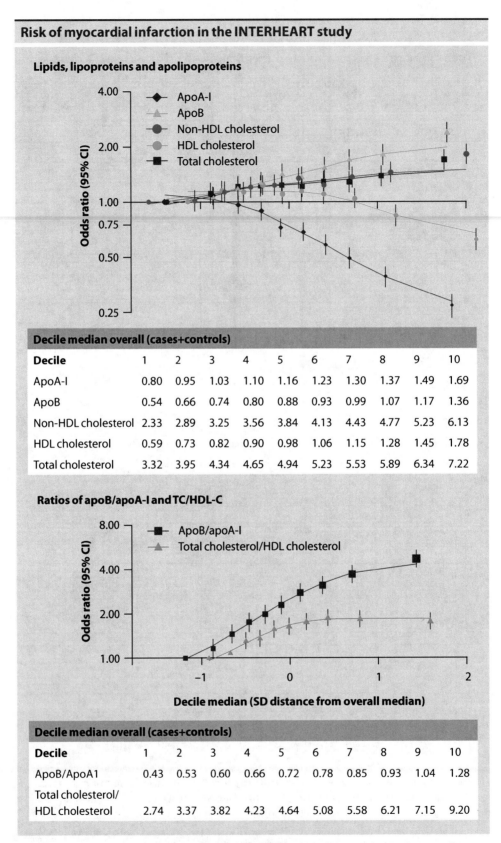

Risk of myocardial infarction in the INTERHEART study

Lipids, lipoproteins and apolipoproteins

Legend:
- ApoA-I
- ApoB
- Non-HDL cholesterol
- HDL cholesterol
- Total cholesterol

Decile median overall (cases+controls)

Decile	1	2	3	4	5	6	7	8	9	10
ApoA-I	0.80	0.95	1.03	1.10	1.16	1.23	1.30	1.37	1.49	1.69
ApoB	0.54	0.66	0.74	0.80	0.88	0.93	0.99	1.07	1.17	1.36
Non-HDL cholesterol	2.33	2.89	3.25	3.56	3.84	4.13	4.43	4.77	5.23	6.13
HDL cholesterol	0.59	0.73	0.82	0.90	0.98	1.06	1.15	1.28	1.45	1.78
Total cholesterol	3.32	3.95	4.34	4.65	4.94	5.23	5.53	5.89	6.34	7.22

Ratios of apoB/apoA-I and TC/HDL-C

Legend:
- ApoB/apoA-I
- Total cholesterol/HDL cholesterol

Decile median (SD distance from overall median)

Decile median overall (cases+controls)

Decile	1	2	3	4	5	6	7	8	9	10
ApoB/ApoA1	0.43	0.53	0.60	0.66	0.72	0.78	0.85	0.93	1.04	1.28
Total cholesterol/HDL cholesterol	2.74	3.37	3.82	4.23	4.64	5.08	5.58	6.21	7.15	9.20

Figure 6.4 Risk of myocardial infarction in the INTERHEART study. Note the doubling scale on the y axis in both part A and part B. Apo, apolipoprotein; HDL-C, high-density lipopraotein cholesterol; TC, total cholesterol. Reproduced with permission from [7].

there is an enormous body of data about cholesterol in epidemiology, clinical diagnosis, risk prediction and choice of management. So far, this is not the case for apolipoproteins. In addition, there are two major recent guidelines dealing with the management and prevention of atherosclerotic CVD, and they focus on the role of cholesterol in this regard (ATP III and euroSCORE).

One disadvantage of the cholesterol-based profile is that blood must be taken in the fasting state because 'meal-sensitive' triglycerides are included in this profile. Another disadvantage is that LDL-C is calculated from three different lipids' levels, increasing the error of the estimate. Because of the great variability of LDL-C, ATP III has recommended three determinations of LDL-C in order to obtain a value that is as true as possible.

Advantages of the apolipoprotein-based lipid profile

In contrast to the cholesterol-based lipid profile, for determination of the apolipoprotein profile blood samples can be taken in the non-fasting state, i.e. at any time during the day and without interruption of daily life. In addition, measurements of the apolipoproteins are internationally standardised. Furthermore, in contrast to LDL-C, apoB is an exact measurement of the number of atherogenic lipoproteins because VLDL, IDL, LDL and Lp(a) contain just one molecule apoB per particle. Finally, the ratio apoB/apoA-I can give insight into the relations between cholesterol entry into and efflux from cells (Figure 4.3).

Currently, a disadvantage of the apolipoprotein-based lipid profile is that so far there are no international guidelines for its use, whether in risk prediction or in management approaches to the prevention and treatment of clinical atherosclerosis, in clinical practice. However, there is no doubt that such guidelines will soon appear in the clinical arena.

Is any single profile best?

It is not always possible to say that one or the other is best for a particular set of circumstances. Both the cholesterol-based and the apolipoprotein-based lipid profiles are good.

In the choice between these two excellent approaches in lipid testing and risk prediction, a linguistic aspect might be worth considering, in that atherosclerosis starts with accumulation of cholesterol in the arterial wall, and statins – the 'wonder drugs' for its treatment – are cholesterol lowering. So there is a an awareness of cholesterol in both the aetiology and the treatment of atherosclerosis, and nowadays this holds true among the general public as well as the medical profession. The current use of a cholesterol-based lipid profile may therefore in itself be facilitating the communication of a number of different aspects of clinical atherosclerosis, including both lipid testing and management.

PART TWO

Lipid management

Chapter 7

Goals of lipid management

Clinical goals of lipid management

The three major clinical goals of lipid management are:

- primary prevention of clinical atherosclerosis,
- secondary prevention of clinical atherosclerosis, and
- identification and treatment of secondary dyslipidaemias.

Other goals of lipid management include prevention of recurrent attacks of pancreatitis in severe hypertriglyceridaemia and resolution of cutaneous and tendinous xanthomata.

Primary prevention of clinical atherosclerosis

Primary prevention of clinical atherosclerosis is the long-term treatment of risk factors believed to be causal for clinical atherosclerosis in patients without evidence of clinical atherosclerosis. Important groups of patients in this respect are patients with genetic dyslipidaemias – FH (type IIA hyperlipidaemia), familial combined hyperlipidaemia, type III hyperlipidaemia – and diabetes mellitus. Primary prevention aims to prevent development of the manifestations of clinical atherosclerosis (Figure 1.1).

Secondary prevention of clinical atherosclerosis

Secondary prevention of clinical atherosclerosis is the long-term treatment of risk factors believed to be causal for clinical atherosclerosis in patients with existing clinical atherosclerosis. Secondary prevention is necessary because patients who already have manifestations of clinical atherosclerosis are at high risk of recurrence of or new manifestations of clinical atherosclerosis. Secondary prevention aims to prevent this.

Prevention and treatment of rare complications of severe dyslipidaemia

Acute pancreatitis

Acute pancreatitis may occur in type V hyperlipidaemia, particularly when fasting triglyceride levels are above 20 mmol/L (1771 mg/dL) although this life-threatening complication does not occur in all subjects with type V hyperlipidaemia. Typically the attacks are recurrent, often monthly. Treatment of the severe hypertriglyceridaemia by a very low-fat diet may diminish intensity and number of attacks. Nicotinic acid in high doses is the treatment of choice normalising the hypertriglyceridaemia and abolishing the attacks.

Xanthomata

Xanthomata, particularly in the form of xanthelasmata, may have a pronounced cosmetic effect impairing the quality of life. In addition both tuberous/eruptive and tendinous xanthomata may interfere with the actions of hands and feet The tuberous ones may disappear after a few months intensive treatment with fibrates or nicotinic acid, tendinous xanthomata are more refractive to lipid-modifying treatment.

Identification and treatment of secondary dyslipidaemias

Secondary dyslipidaemias may be caused by many underlying diseases, as listed in Figure 7.1. The lipoprotein changes in a number of them are shown in Figure 7.2, increased VLDL and LDL, as well as decreased HDL, may be present.

In clinical practice, diabetes mellitus, metabolic syndrome, hypothyroidism and kidney diseases are the conditions most often associated with dyslipidaemia. Treatment of these diseases may alleviate or even 'cure' the dyslipidaemia.

Lipid goals in lipid management

The goals of lipid management are:

- normalisation of lipid levels in dyslipidaemia,
- achievement of guideline-specified lipid levels for patients in defined risk categories,

- achievement of desirable levels of lipid risk factors, and
- long-term control of the lipid profile response to treatment, including attention to adverse reactions.

Lipid and lipoprotein targets

Of the lipid risk factors listed in Figure 1.6, LDL-C is the most important one to modify when aiming to prevent clinical atherosclerosis. The two major reasons for this are the high atherogenicity of LDL and the internationally and well-documented diminished occurrence of manifestations of clinical atherosclerosis when treatment reduces LDL-C.

Secondary dyslipidaemias	
Endocrine	Diabetes mellitus
	Thyroid disease
	Pituitary disease
	Pregnancy
	Metabolic syndrome
Hepatic	Cholestatis
	Hepatocellular disease
	Cholelithiasis
Hyperuricaemic	Gout
Iatrogenic	Antiretroviral agents
	Beta-blockers
	Microsomal enzyme-inducing agents (e.g. griseofulvin, phenobarbitol, phenytoin)
	Retinoic acid derivatives
	Steroid hormones
	Thiazide diuretics
Immune	Myeloma
	Macrogobulinaemia
	Systemic lupus erythematosus
Miscellaneous	Glycogen storage disease
	Lipodystrophies
Nutritional	Alcoholism
	Anorexia nervosa
	Obesity
Renal	Chronic renal failure
	Nephrotic syndrome

Figure 7.1 Secondary dyslipidaemias.

It is also important in this context to consider the other lipid risk factors, particularly high levels of triglycerides and Lp(a) and low levels of protective HDL. In most trials, intensive, maximal lowering of LDL has reduced CHD events by 25–40%. By implication, coronary events were not prevented in 60–75% of high-risk patients, despite aggressive LDL-reducing treatment. This level of 'residual risk' is unacceptably high. Thus, to improve the prognosis of high-risk patients and reduce residual risk, the other major lipid risk factors should be candidates for lipid-lowering management. Abnormal levels should be addressed when possible and non-lipid risk factors should also be dealt with.

Cornerstones of lipid management

The two cornerstones of lipid management are improvement of lifestyle and pharmacological treatment.

Improvement of lifestyle

Improvement of lifestyle consists of three steps:
- dietary recommendations,
- physical activity recommendations, and
- cessation of smoking and other substance abuses

Lipoprotein levels in secondary dislipidaemias			
Cause	VLDL	LDL	HDL
Diabetes type 1	↑	– or ↓	– or ↑
Diabetes type 2	↑↑	↑	↓
Metabolic syndrome	↑	–	↓
Hypothyroidism	↑	↑↑	↑
Pregnancy	↑	↑	↑
Obesity	↑	– or ↑	↓
Alcohol	↑	– or ↑	↑
Nephrotic syndrome	↑	↑↑	– or ↓
Chronic renal failure	↑	–	↓
Cholestasis	–	↑↑*	↓
Hepatocellular disease	↑†	–	↓
Hyperuricaemia	↑	–	↓

Figure 7.2 Lipoprotein levels in secondary dislipidaemias. HDL, high-density lipoprotein; LDL, low-density lipoprotein; VLDL, very low-density lipoprotein. *Lipoprotein X. †Intermediate density lipoprotein. Modified from [23].

The major effect of lifestyle measures on dyslipidaemia is of course mainly obtained by dietary changes. The other two steps, particularly smoking cessation, are of great importance for prevention of manifestations of clinical atherosclerosis but they have only marginal effects on the lipid profile.

Pharmacological treatment

Pharmacological treatment has to be considered in when improvements in lifestyle have not resulted in a satisfactory lipid profile. The choice and dosage of pharmacotherapies for lipid management are described in detail in Chapter 10. Statins are indisputably the leading, most universally used lipid-modifying drug class, not only because of their effect on the lipid profile (mainly a lowering of LDL-C) but also because of their well-documented beneficial clinical effects on prevention of clinical atherosclerosis. There are, however, other lipid-modifying drug classes that have their own specific indications, such as reducing high triglyceride levels and raising low HDL levels of HDL; these are described in detail in Chapter 10.

Chapter 8

Cholesterol lowering and prevention of CHD

The first steps
The Coronary Primary Prevention Trial (CPPT)

In the 1950s two potent cholesterol-lowering drugs appeared, nicotinic acid (niacin) in high doses for lipid modification (far exceeding its dose when used as a vitamin), and cholestyramine, a bile acid sequestrant. Both were effective in humans, had a dose–response effect on cholesterol levels and were difficult to manage, nicotinic acid because of its side-effect of facial flushing and cholestyramine because of the large doses required and because of its interference with the absorption of many other drugs. However, many studies with these drugs proved their excellent effects on high plasma cholesterol levels.

Furthermore, with cholestyramine a new and important clinical facet was introduced into cholesterol-lowering trials: not only measuring the effect on lipid levels but also (and most importantly) assessing the effect on the occurrence of clinical atherosclerosis. In a large trial, the LRC-CPPT, nearly 4,000 hypercholesterolaemic men without clinical atherosclerosis were randomly assigned to cholestyramine 24 g/day or placebo for an average of 7 years. Total cholesterol and LDL-C were lowered by 13 and 20%, respectively. The risk for CHD decreased by 19% in this pivotal study, but mortality was unaffected [24]. CPPT, published in 1984, was the first double-blind placebo-controlled trial showing unambiguously that cholesterol lowering in high-risk men significantly reduced the risk of CHD.

The Scandinavian Simvastatin Survival Study (4S)

With CPPT a first step had been taken towards investigating the clinical effects of cholesterol lowering and the door had been opened on the enormous and rapidly growing field of lipid management for prevention of clinical atherosclerosis. The next step in management of high cholesterol came in the early 1990s with the 4S secondary prevention trial [25]. This landmark study showed that reduction of cholesterol with a statin (simvastatin) led to significant reductions in the occurrence of new manifestations of clinical atherosclerosis and, most importantly, in total mortality. 4S is described in more detail below.

The statin era

The beneficial effects observed in 4S – significant reductions in the occurrence of manifestations of clinical atherosclerosis and CHD and total mortality – were soon confirmed by other clinical trials of statins (Figure 8.1). The doors to the statin era had been opened.

Beginning of the statin era

The statins had been discovered by Akira Endo, a Japanese microbiologist working for the company Sankyo. In the beginning of the 1970s Endo began to search for microbial metabolites that might inhibit HMG-CoA reductase, the rate-limiting enzyme in the synthesis of cholesterol from acetate.

Endo's original stroke of genius was the simple idea that in order to lower plasma cholesterol one should inhibit the hepatic synthesis of cholesterol instead of trying to inhibit gastrointestinal absorption of cholesterol and/or bile acids. In their first publication, Endo and co-workers described the discovery and isolation of compactin (ML 236 B), the original statin, isolated from *Penicillium citrinum* [30]. They showed that compactin was a potent inhibitor of HMG-CoA reductase and, as a result, had hypocholesterolaemic effects as expected. This report was soon followed by the first reports of human studies showing that treatment with compactin resulted in significant lowering of LDL-C in patients with FH [31].

Endo and investigators at the Merck company then isolated lovastatin, which became the first statin to be licensed in USA. Other statins were by then in the pipeline for cholesterol lowering, for example pravastatin (derived from compactin), simvastatin (derived from lovastatin), atorvastatin (the world's highest selling drug) and rosuvastatin (a very potent statin).

In 2008 Endo was awarded the prestigious Lasker-De Bakey Clinical Medical Research Award for his discovery of the statins.

Early ground-breaking statin trials

At the end of the 1990s five landmark trials, headed by the 4S trial, three in secondary prevention and two in primary prevention, were

Landmark studies in cholesterol lowering with statins

	4S [25]	CARE [26]	LIPID [27]	WOSCOPS [28]	AFCAPS/ TexCAPS [29]
Primary or secondary prevention	2°	2°	2°	1°	1°
No. of patients	4444	4159	9014	6595	6605
Women (%)	18	14	17	0	15
Mean age (years)	59	59	62	55	58
Mean cholesterol level:					
mmol/L	6.8	5.4	5.7	7.0	5.7
mg/dL	263	208	220	271	220
Reduction (%) by statins of:					
TC levels	25	20	18	20	18
LDL-C levels	35	28	25	26	25
CHD events in men	30	18	26	30	37
CHD events in women	42	42	11 (ns)	–	47
Stroke events	29	31	20	10 (ns)	–
CHD mortality	41	19 (ns)	23	27 (ns)*	27 (ns)*
Study drug	Simvastatin 40 mg	Pravastatin 40 mg	Pravastatin 40 mg	Pravastatin 40 mg	Lovastatin 20–40 mg
Nephrotic syndrome	↑	↑↑	– or ↓		
Chronic renal failure	↑	–	↓		
Cholestasis	–	↑↑*	↓		
Hepatocellular disease	↑†	–	↓		
Hyperuricaemia	↑	–	↓		

Figure 8.1 Landmark studies in cholesterol lowering with statins. CHD, coronary heart disease; ns, not significant (all other changes were statistically significant). *In these two primary prevention studies, the number of deaths from CHD was too low (90 and 26, respectively) to allow meaningful interpretation.

published that all showed that cholesterol lowering by statins in high-risk subjects was associated with a significantly decreased risk of clinical atherosclerosis (Figure 8.1). The statin dose was similar in all trial, 20–40 mg/day. The lowering of total-C was on average 18–25% and that of LDL-C 25–35%. There was a significant reduction in CHD events among men in all five studies and among women in three of the four studies that included women. There was also a reduction in the number of strokes. CHD mortality had been reduced by 19–41% and total mortality by 8–21% in these trials. The concordance in the results of these landmark trials is eloquent: statin treatment not only lowers plasma cholesterol but also reduces morbidity and mortality from clinical atherosclerosis.

These five landmark trials were followed by a number of other studies on the clinical outcomes of statin treatment in the prevention of clinical atherosclerosis. The results of some of the major early trials are summarised in Figure 8.2. Foremost of these to start reporting results were two large statin trials, the secondary prevention British HPS study [32] and the primary prevention trial JUPITER from the USA [33].

British HPS – a major ground-breaking statin trial

The 4S trial was a major breakthrough in the cardiovascular protection via cholesterol lowering with statins. Subsequently, due to its large size and careful planning, HPS significantly increased our understanding of preventive lipid management using statins in patients with clinical atherosclerosis and diabetes. HPS comprised 20,000 subjects, including 5000 females, age 40–80 years, with either clinical atherosclerosis or diabetes, randomised to 40 mg/day of simvastatin or placebo during a planned 5-year treatment period.

Lipid results

The mean basal non-fasting cholesterol concentrations (mmol/L) were: total-C 5.9 (228 mg/dL), LDL-C 3.4 (131 mg/dL), HDL-C 1.1 (43 mg/dL). The treatment with simvastatin reduced LDL-C by 1 mmol/L (39 mg/dL) in the intention-to-treat analysis and by 1.5 mmol/L (58 mg/dL) for those actually taking the statin during the trial.

Mortality

Total mortality was decreased by 13% in the statin group (Figure 8.3), mainly due to a decrease in vascular causes. Death rates due to non-vascular causes were similar in the placebo and treatment group (Figure 8.3).

Vascular events

The rate of non-fatal myocardial infarction was reduced by nearly 40% in the simvastatin group, as shown in Figure 8.4, which also shows a significant reduction in other major cardiovascular events.

Beneficial effects on clinical atherosclerosis in different patient categories

The large size and long duration of HPS made it possible to evaluate the effects in different patient populations. Treatment with simvastatin was found to be effective in significantly reducing major cardiovascular events in:

- primary as well as secondary prevention of clinical atherosclerosis,
- older as well as younger subjects,
- women as well as men,
- patients with and without diabetes,
- those with LDL-C below as well as above 3 mmol/L (116 mg/dL), and
- those with total-C below as well as above 5 mmol/L (193 mg/dL).

Myopathy, an adverse effect of statin treatment, occurred in 0.01% of the statin-treated patients.

JUPITER – a major ground-breaking primary prevention statin trial

JUPITER comprised 18,000 apparently healthy male (age >50 years) and female (age >60 years) subjects, 40% and 60 %, respectively, with LDL-C <3.4 mmol/L (130 mg/dL) and a hs-CRP >2.0 mg/L. After a run-in period the allocated subjects were randomised to receive placebo or rosuvastatin 20 mg per day. The JUPITER trial was stopped after a median follow-up time of 1.9 years due to recommendations of the Data Safety Monitoring Committee based on the pronounced reduction of the number of new cardiovascular events in the group treated with rosuvastatin compared to placebo. There had been 251 events of the

Summary of major statin trials

Study	Follow-up (years)	Patients	Drug	Dose (mg/day)
4S [25]	5.4	4444 adults with angina or prior MI	Simvastatin	40
LIPID [27]	6.1	9014 adults with prior MI or UA (DM 9%, HTN 42%, obese 18%, smokers 10%)	Pravastatin	40
CARE [26]	5	4159 adults with prior MI	Pravastatin	40
HPS [32]	5	20,536 adults with CHD, AD, or D	Simvastatin	40
ALERT [34]	5.1	2102 renal transplant patients (DM 19%, HTN 76%, smokers 19%)	Fluvastatin	40
ALLHAT-LLT [35]	4.8	10,355 adults with HTN (CHD 14%, DM 35%, smokers 23%)	Pravastatin	40
PROSPER [36]	3.2	5804 adults age 70–82 years (CHD 13%, DM 11%, PAD 7%, smokers 26%, TIA 11%, vascular disease 44%)	Pravastatin	40
ASCOT-LLA [37]	3.3	10,305 adults with HTN and ≥3 RFs (CVA/TIA 10%, DM 25%, PAD 5%, smokers 32%)	Atorvastatin	10
LIPS [38]	3.9	1677 adults post-PCI (DM 14%, prior MI 44%, PAD 6%, smokers 25%)	Fluvastatin	80
SPARCL [39]	4.9	4731 adults with prior CVA or TIA and no CHD (DM 17%, HTN 62%, smokers 19%)	Atorvastatin	80
CARDS [40]	3.9	2838 adults with DM + 1 RF and no CVD (HTN 84%, obese 37%, smokers 23%)	Atorvastatin	10
WOSCOPS [41]	4.9	6595 men with no CHD (DM 1%, HTN 15%, smokers 44%)	Pravastatin	40
AFCAPS/TexCAPS [42]	5.2	6605 adults without CHD, HDL C <35mg/dL in men, <40 in women (HTN 22%, smokers 13%)	Lovastatin	20"40

AD, arterial disease; CHD, coronary heart disease; CVA, cerebrovascular accident; CVD, cardiovascular disease; D, diabetes; DM, diabetes mellitus; HDL-C, high-density lipoprotein cholesterol; HTN, hypertension; LDL-C, low-density lipoprotein cholesterol; MI, myocardial infarction; ns, not significant; PAD, peripheral artery disease; PCI, percutaneous coronary intervention; RF, risk factor; TIA, transient ischaemic attack.

Figure 8.2 Summary of major statin trials. All were placebo-controlled, randomised, double-blind and had clinical events as their endpoints. Adapted from [43].

| LDL-C start | | LDL-C end | | | |
mmol/L	mg/dL	mmol/L	mg/dL	Reduction (%)	CHD reduction (%)
4.9	190	3.0	117	35	34
3.9	150	2.9	112	25	24
3.6	139	2.5	98	32	24
3.4	132	2.3	89	32	27
4.1	159	2.8	108	32	35
3.8	146	2.7	105	17	9 (ns)
3.8	147	2.8	107	27	19
3.4	133	2.3	87	35	36
3.4	132	2.5	96	27	31 (*p*=0.07)
3.4	132	1.9	73	45	35
3.1	118	2.0	78	31	35
5.0	192	3.7	142	26	31
3.9	150	3.0	115	25	40

primary endpoint (major cardiovascular events) in the placebo group but only 142 events in the rosuvastatin treated group, the hazard ratio for rosuvastatin was 0.56 (95% CI 0.46–0.69, p <0.00001).

Rosuvastatin reduced LDL concentration by 50% and the levels of hs-CRP by 37%. The time course for the occurrence of four major groups of clinical events (shown in Figure 8.5) was: 1) primary end point (major cardiovascular events); 2) combination of myocardial infarction, stroke and cardiovascular death; 3) revascularisation and unstable angina; and 4) death from any cause. For all groups the treatment with rosuvastatin had significantly reduced the incidence of events. With time the reduction of events by treatment with rosuvastatin becomes more and more pronounced compared to placebo. The beneficial effects of rosuvastatin on cardiovascular events as well as on total mortality were equally significant for males as for females, for younger as well as for

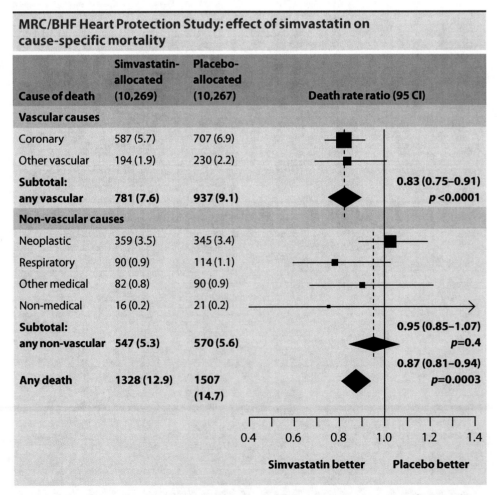

Figure 8.3 MRC/BHF Heart Protection Study: effect of simvastatin on cause-specific mortality.
Reproduced with permission from Heart Protection Study Collaborative Group. Lancet 2002;360:7–22.

older subjects, for smokers as for non-smokers, for hypertensives as for normotensives, for those with high as for those with normal BMI.

A detailed analysis [43] of the results of JUPITER showed that the participants who had obtained an LDL-C <1.8 mmol/L (70 mg/dL), the goal for high risk persons set by ATP III (see Chapter 9), had a 55% reduction in cardiovascular events. Rosuvastatin had induced an even more pronounced reduction of 65% in patients who had obtained an LDL-C of 1.8 mmol/l as well as a hs-CRP <2 mg/L in response to the treatment. The superior beneficial effect of rosuvastatin on LDL-C as well as on HDL-C compared to other statins was shown in the STELLAR trial (see Chapter 11).

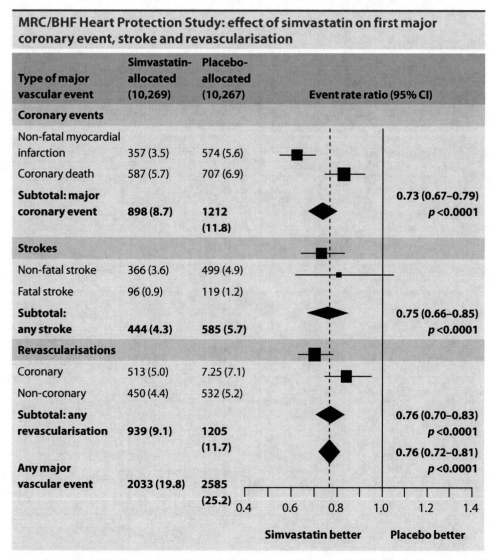

Type of major vascular event	Simvastatin-allocated (10,269)	Placebo-allocated (10,267)	Event rate ratio (95% CI)
Coronary events			
Non-fatal myocardial infarction	357 (3.5)	574 (5.6)	
Coronary death	587 (5.7)	707 (6.9)	
Subtotal: major coronary event	**898 (8.7)**	**1212 (11.8)**	0.73 (0.67–0.79) *p* <0.0001
Strokes			
Non-fatal stroke	366 (3.6)	499 (4.9)	
Fatal stroke	96 (0.9)	119 (1.2)	
Subtotal: any stroke	**444 (4.3)**	**585 (5.7)**	0.75 (0.66–0.85) *p* <0.0001
Revascularisations			
Coronary	513 (5.0)	7.25 (7.1)	
Non-coronary	450 (4.4)	532 (5.2)	
Subtotal: any revascularisation	**939 (9.1)**	**1205 (11.7)**	0.76 (0.70–0.83) *p* <0.0001
Any major vascular event	**2033 (19.8)**	**2585 (25.2)**	0.76 (0.72–0.81) *p* <0.0001

MRC/BHF Heart Protection Study: effect of simvastatin on first major coronary event, stroke and revascularisation

0.4 0.6 0.8 1.0 1.2 1.4

Simvastatin better   Placebo better

Figure 8.4 MRC/BHF Heart Protection Study: effect of simvastatin on first major coronary event, stroke and revascularisation (defined prospectively as 'major vascular events'). Reproduced with permission from [32].

Cumulative incidence of four groups of clinical events in the rosuvastatin and placebo groups

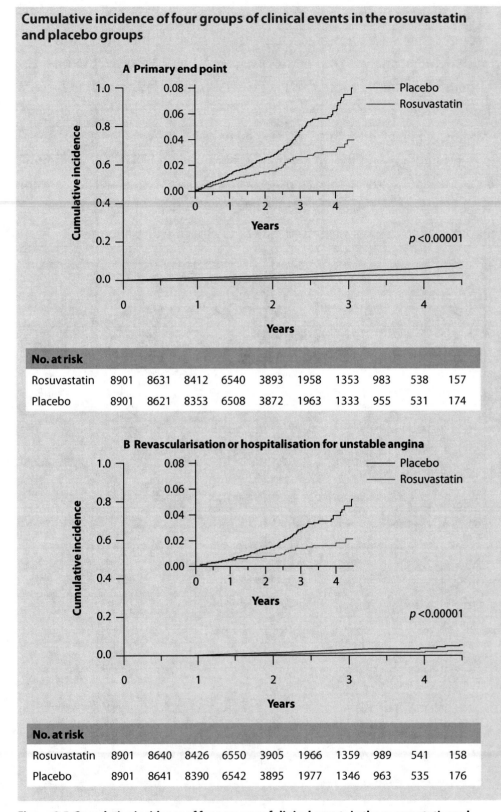

Figure 8.5 Cumulative incidence of four groups of clinical events in the rosuvastatin and placebo groups. Reproduced with permission from [33].

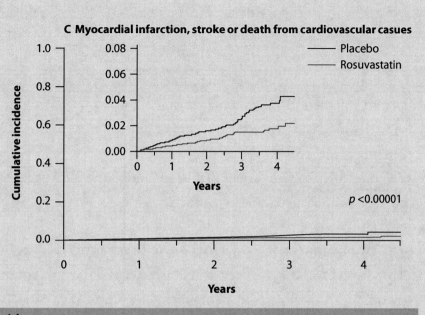

C Myocardial infarction, stroke or death from cardiovascular casues

Cumulative incidence vs Years

p <0.00001

No. at risk										
Rosuvastatin	8901	8643	8437	6571	3921	1979	1370	998	545	159
Placebo	8901	8633	8381	6542	3918	1992	1365	979	547	181

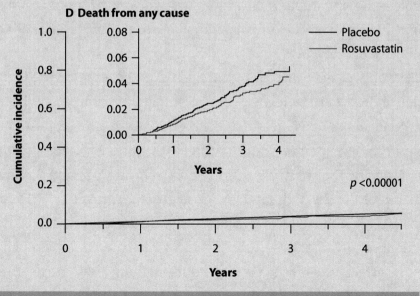

D Death from any cause

Cumulative incidence vs Years

p <0.00001

No. at risk										
Rosuvastatin	8901	8847	8787	6999	4312	2268	1602	1192	676	227
Placebo	8901	8852	8775	6987	4319	2295	1614	1196	681	246

Two important aspects of cholesterol lowering

The five statin landmark trials, the HPS and several other subsequent statin trials (Figure 8.2) have conveyed the same general message that cholesterol lowering by statins will reduce the occurrence of manifestations of clinical atherosclerosis, including reduction of mortality. These results naturally led to two important questions:

- Is the degree of cholesterol lowering of importance for the clinical outcome?
- Which is the best measure of LDL-C in lipid management for the prevention of clinical atherosclerosis?

Degree of cholesterol lowering – the lower the better?

The TNT (Treat to New Target) trial was a secondary prevention trial designed to test this question by comparing the clinical effects of intensive cholesterol lowering using a high dose of atorvastatin (80 mg/day) with the results of a low dose (10 mg/day) [45]. TNT comprised 10,001 patients with LDL-C <3.4 mmol/L (<130 mg/dL). The design was a double-blind, randomised treatment with the two doses of atorvastatin planned for 5 years. The primary endpoint was the appearance of a major cardiovascular event.

The effects over time for LDL-C and total-C are shown in Figure 8.6, which shows that the levels were constant over time after the initial reduction and that, as expected, the higher dose of atorvastatin reduced cholesterol levels more than did the lower dose. The mean values for LDL-C during the study were 2.0 mmol/L (77 mg/dL) and 2.6 mmol/L (101 mg/dL) in the high- and low-dose groups, respectively. There was also a decrease of triglycerides but no significant change in HDL-C with either dose.

The effect on various manifestations of clinical atherosclerosis are shown in Figure 8.7. The patterns are the same for all four manifestations, with a reduction of events which was more pronounced in the high-dose group. Haemorrhagic strokes occurred in 16 and 17 cases in the high- and low-dose groups, respectively, and death from cancer in 85 and 75 groups, respectively ($p=0.42$). Myopathy was reported in 241 and 234 patients, respectively, and rhabdomyolysis in 2 and 3 patients, respectively. Elevated alanine or aspartate aminotransferase occurred in 60 patients in the high-dose group and in 9 in the low-dose group (p <0.001).

A compilation of results from six secondary prevention trials with statins is displayed in Figure 8.8 [45]. This illustrates the presence of an impressive linear relationship between the lowering of LDL-C and the occurrence of events of clinical atherosclerosis, a strong argument for 'the lower the LDL-C, the better' in the use of statins in the prevention of clinical atherosclerosis.

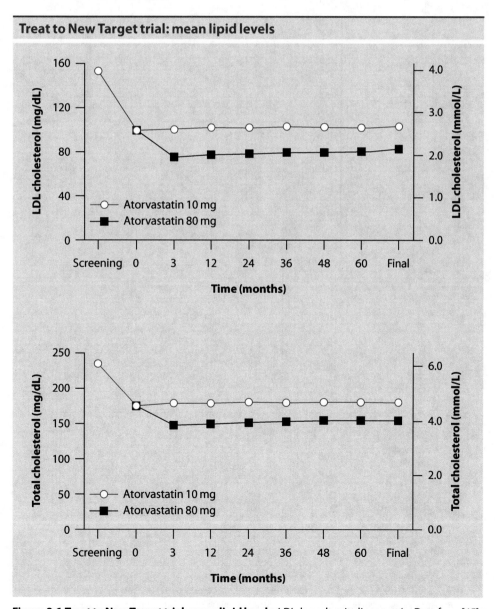

Figure 8.6 Treat to New Target trial: mean lipid levels. LDL, low-density lipoprotein. Data from [45].

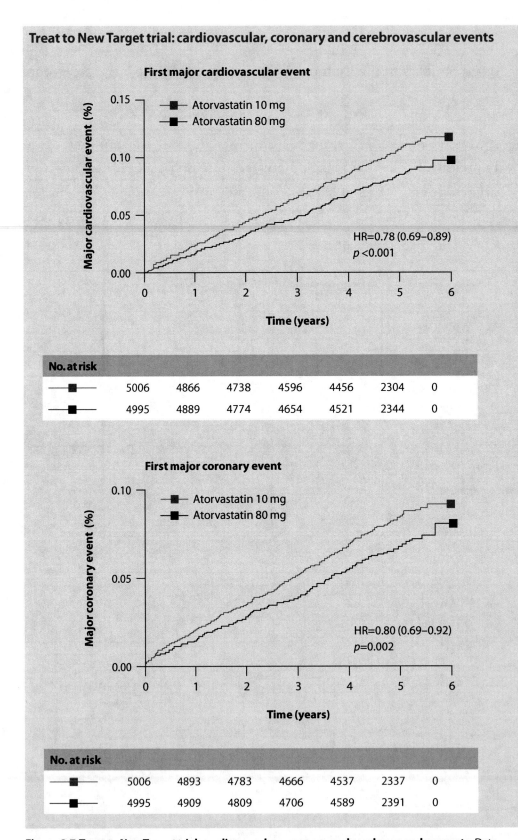

Figure 8.7 Treat to New Target trial: cardiovascular, coronary and cerebrovascular events. Data are cumulative incidence. HD, coronary heart disease; MI, myocardial infarction. Data from [45].

Nonfatal MI or death from CHD

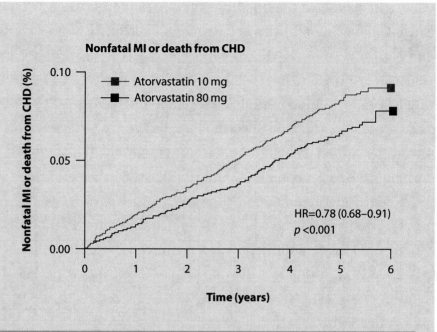

No. at risk							
▣—	5006	4693	4792	4670	4539	2361	0
■—	4995	4911	4812	4715	4596	2395	0

First fatal or nonfatal stroke

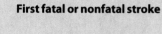

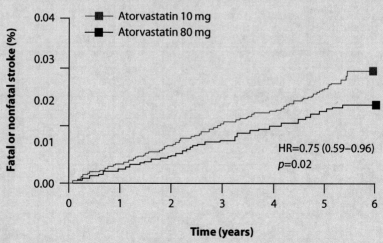

No. at risk							
▣—	5006	4937	4859	4761	4663	2447	0
■—	4995	4937	4862	4771	4684	2451	0

Further evidence for this linear relationship between the degree of LDL-C lowering and the occurrence of cardiovascular events has been obtained in other recent reports. CTT (Cholesterol Treatment Trialists) performed a meta-analysis on the efficacy of cholesterol lowering based on 14 randomised trials comprising nearly 100,000 statin-treated patients [46]. Published in 2005, this study collected data from 14 trials it defined as being 'properly randomised'. On average LDL-C was reduced by 1.1 mmol/L (42 mg/dL) in these trials and there was a 19% proportional reduction of coronary mortality (p <0.0001). Major vascular events were reduced by about 20% per mmol/L (39 mg/dL) reduction in LDL-C, and there was a significant trend for a linear relation between the absolute reduction of LDL-C and the reduction of both major coronary events and major vascular events (Figure 8.9). Once again, 'the lower the better' held true.

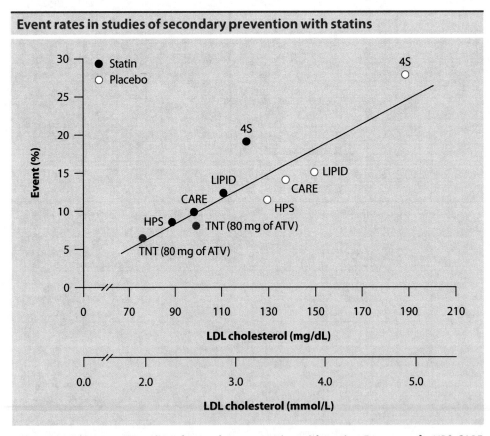

Figure 8.8 Event rates in studies of secondary prevention with statins. Event rates for HPS, CARE and LIPID are for death from CHD and nonfatal myocardial infarction. Event rates for 4S and TNT also include resuscitation after cardiac arrest. ATV, atorvastatin; CARE, Cholesterol and Recurrent Events Trial [26]; HPS, Heart Protection Study [32]; LIPID, Long-term Intervention with Pravastatin in Ischaemic Disease [27]; 4S, Scandinavian Simvastatin Survival Study [25]. Data from [45].

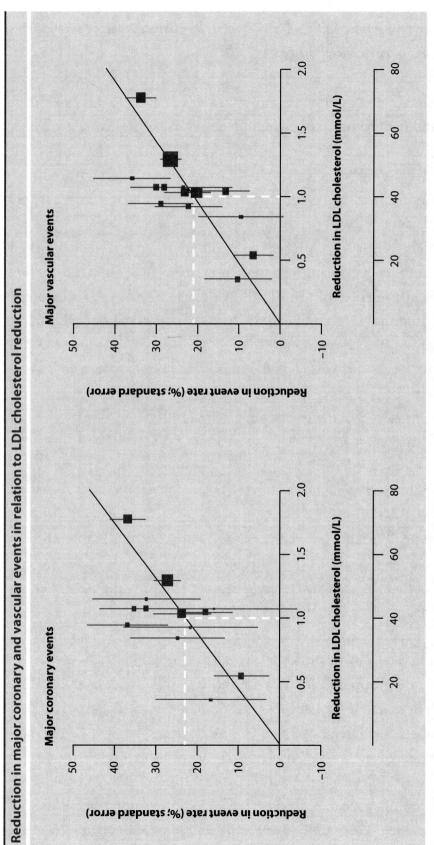

Figure 8.9 Reduction in major coronary and vascular events in relation to LDL cholesterol reduction. Each square represents a single trial plotted against mean absolute LDL cholesterol reduction at 1 year, with vertical lines above and below corresponding to one standard error of unweighted event rate reduction. Trials are plotted in order of magnitude of difference in LDL cholesterol difference at 1 year. Data from a meta-analysis of 14 trials comprising nearly 100,000 patients [46].

Which measures of LDL-C predict the clinical outcome best in cholesterol-lowering trials?

The ultimate goal for cholesterol lowering is of course to achieve the most effective prevention of manifestations of clinical atherosclerosis. Hence the facility to predict the outcome in the clinical setting is of the greatest importance. With regard to use of LDL-C in prediction the pre-treatment level and relative or absolute treatment-induced reduction of LDL-C have been evaluated and discussed as measures for such predictions.

A major study comprising over 150,000 participants and published in 2010 has reported results of a meta-regression analysis of the relation of different measures of LDL-C relative to the risk of CAD. The study was based on 20 large-scale trials of statins versus either placebo or usual care [47]. The relation of the following five measures of LDL-C to the two endpoints CAD and all-cause mortality, respectively, were evaluated:

- baseline LDL-C in the treatment group: LDLRx
- absolute change in LDL-C in the treatment group: ΔLDLBaseline-Final
- percentage change in LDL-C in the treatment group: %ΔLDLBaseline-Final
- absolute difference between achieved in-trial LDL-C in the control vs treatment group: ΔLDLControl-Rx
- percentage difference between achieved LDL-C in the control vs treatment group: %ΔLDLControl-Rx

The main results are shown in Figure 8.10. For all RCTs and for RCTs without active comparators the absolute reduction in LDL-C was the strongest determinant of CAD risk and was independent of baseline LDL-C. For mortality, however, baseline LDL-C was the strongest predictor of risk, followed by the absolute decrease of LDL-C. The percentage decrease of LDL-C had no significant influence on the risk of mortality. In conclusion the authors stated 'these findings underscore the *primacy of absolute reductions in LDL cholesterol* in the design and interpretation of RCTs of lipid-lowering therapies and in framing treatment recommendations'.

Summary

The available evidence suggests that:

- **a low LDL-C/total-C** ('the lower, the better'), out of all measures focussing on LDL, gives the best protection against the occurrence of clinical atherosclerosis, and

- **the absolute reduction of LDL-C**, rather than the percentage reduction, is the best predictor of the clinical outcome of LDL treatment.

	RCTs without active comparators		All RCTs	
Variable	**β per SD increase**	**p**	**β per SD increase**	**p**
Coronary artery disease, lnOR$_{CAD}$				
Baseline LDL$_{Rx}$	−0.045	0.320	−0.083	0.014
ΔLDL$_{Baseline-Final}$	−0.091	0.052	−0.082	0.029
%ΔLDL$_{Baseline-Final}$	−0.063	0.221	−0.062	0.143
ΔLDL$_{Control-Rx}$	−0.108	<0.001	−0.129	<0.001
%ΔLDL$_{Control-Rx}$	−0.095	0.030	−0.127	<0.001
All-cause mortality, lnOR$_{Mortality}$				
Baseline LDL$_{Rx}$	−0.065	0.081	−0.067	0.022
ΔLDL$_{Baseline-Final}$	−0.018	0.686	−0.021	0.511
%ΔLDL$_{Baseline-Final}$	0.020	0.581	0.002	0.941
ΔLDL$_{Control-Rx}$	−0.030	0.397	−0.055	0.041
%ΔLDL$_{Control-Rx}$	0	0.993	−0.030	0.297

Figure 8.10 Meta-regression for coronary artery disease or death as a function of lipid measures or trial duration. Data are for 20 trials comprising over 150,000 patients. RCTs, randomised controlled trials; β, standardised regression coefficient; Δ, change; LDL, low-density lipoprotein; Rx, treatment group. Adapted with permission from [47].

Chapter 9

Cholesterol goals in current guidelines

LDL-C is the primary target for lipid management. There are four major guidelines:

1. ATP III of NCEP [11,12]
2. European guidelines on CVD [10]
3. British guidelines on prevention of CVD [48]
4. NICE clinical guideline 67 [49]

They unanimously recommend reduction of LDL-C, the major lipid risk factor for clinical atherosclerosis, as the first step in lipid management in primary as well as secondary prevention. However, the lipid goals and the descriptions of the practical approach to reaching the goals varies considerably among these guidelines.

The intensity of the lipid management to be prescribed depends primarily on the patient's total risk for clinical atherosclerosis, evaluated as described in Chapters 5 and 6. The three major factors that determine this risk are:

- presence of CHD and so-called CHD equivalents, i.e. other manifestations of clinical atherosclerosis,
- presence of diabetes, and
- a 20% 10-year risk for CHD (see Chapter 6).

Goals for LDL-C according to ATP III guidelines with proposed modifications

The latest recommendations from NCEP-ATP III about treatment goals for LDL-C and LDL-C thresholds for initiation of treatment are given in Figure 9.1. The major novelty in this recommendation [12], compared with the previous ATP III recommendations [11], is the inclusion of the new optimal LDL-C goal of 1.8 mmol/L (70 mg/dL) for very high risk persons. The underlying reason for this new level, which is substantially lower than earlier goals for LDL-C, is that recent clinical trials have provided greater support for more intensive LDL-lowering, as described above.

Goals for LDL-C according to other guidelines

The European [10], British [50] and NICE [51] guidelines have all defined the goal for LDL-C in high-risk patients as 2.0 mmol/L (80 mg/dL); the European guideline also gives 2.5 mmol/L (96 mg/dL) as an option. Correspondingly, the goal for total-C is set at 4.0–4.5 mmol/L (155–175 mg/dL).

(See opposite) Figure 9.1 ATP III LDL-C goals and thresholds for therapeutic lifestyle changes (TLCs) and drug therapy. Data shown are for different risk categories and based on evidence from recent clinical trials. C, cholesterol; CHD, coronary heart disease; LDL, low-density lipoprotein; HDL, high-density lipoprotein. Adapted from [12].

ATP III LDL-C goals and thresholds for therapeutic lifestyle changes and drug therapy

Risk category	LDL-C goal		Initiate TLC		Consider drug therapy**	
	mmol/L	mg/dL	mmol/L	mg/dL	mmol/L	mg/dL
High risk: CHD* or CHD risk equivalents† (10-year risk >20%)	<2.6 (optional goal: <1.8)¶	<100 (optional goal: <70)¶	≥2.6††	≥100††	≥2.6‡‡ (<2.6: consider drug options)**	≥100‡‡ (<100: consider drug options)**
Moderately high risk: ≥2 risk factors‡ (10-year risk 10% to 20%)§	<3.4	<130**	≥3.4††	≥130††	≥3.4 (2.6–3.3: consider drug options)§§	≥130 (100–129: consider drug options)§§
Moderate risk: ≥2 risk factors (10-year risk <10%)§	<3.4	<130	≥3.4	≥130	≥4.1	≥160
Lower risk: 0–1 risk factor§	<4.1	<160	≥4.1	≥160	≥4.9 (4.1–4.9: LDL-lowering drug optional)	≥190 (160–189: LDL-lowering drug optional)

*CHD includes history of myocardial infarction, unstable angina, stable angina, coronary artery procedures (angioplasty or bypass surgery) or evidence of clinically significant myocardial ischaemia. †CHD risk equivalents include clinical manifestations of non-coronary forms of atherosclerotic disease (peripheral arterial disease, abdominal aortic aneurysm, and carotid artery disease [transient ischaemic attacks or stroke of carotid origin or >50% obstruction of a carotid artery]), diabetes, and ≥2 risk factors with 10-year risk for hard CHD >20%. ‡Risk factors include cigarette smoking, hypertension (blood pressure ≥140/90 mmHg or on antihypertensive medication), low HDL-C (<1.0 mmol/L, <40 mg/dL), family history of premature CHD (CHD in male first-degree relative <55 years of age; CHD in female first-degree relative <65 years of age), and age (men ≥45 years; women ≥55 years). §Electronic 10-year risk calculators are available at www.nhlbi.nih.gov/guidelines/cholesterol. Almost all people with zero or 1 risk factor have a 10-year risk <10%, and 10-year risk assessment in people with ≤1 risk factor is thus not necessary. ¶Very high risk favours the optional LDL-C goal of <1.8 mmol/L (<70 mg/dL), and in patients with high triglycerides, non–HDL-C <2.6 mmol/L (<100 mg/dL). **Optional LDL-C goal <100 mg/dL. ††Any person at high risk or moderately high risk who has lifestyle-related risk factors (e.g., obesity, physical inactivity, elevated triglyceride, low HDL-C or metabolic syndrome) is a candidate for TLC to modify these risk factors regardless of LDL-C level. ‡‡If baseline LDL-C is <2.6 mmol/L (<100 mg/dL), institution of an LDL-lowering drug is a therapeutic option on the basis of available clinical trial results. If a high-risk person has high triglycerides or low HDL-C, combining a fibrate or nicotinic acid with an LDL-lowering drug can be considered. §§For moderately high-risk persons, when LDL-C level is 2.6–3.4 mmol/L (100–129 mg/dL), at baseline or on lifestyle therapy, initiation of an LDL-lowering drug to achieve an LDL-C level <2.6 mmol/L (<100 mg/dL) is a therapeutic option on the basis of available clinical trial results.

Chapter 10

Lipid management in clinical practice

Improvements of lifestyle

An improvement of lifestyle is always the first step in lipid management and should always be continued and checked as long as the patient is under supervision for lipid management. This is emphasised by all guidelines and is called TLC by ATP III.

General aspects

Important general aspects of life style improvement are cessation of smoking, change of a sedentary life style by recommendations about regular exercise, moderation of alcohol intake and body weight reduction (if necessary) with special attention to the high-risk abdominal obesity. Improvement of these aspects of life style will reduce the risk of clinical atherosclerosis, and may also contribute to amendments of the lipid profile. They are easy to recommend, however not always easy to accomplish for the patient or the doctor.

Dietary recommendations for lipid management

Several components of the diet may influence the plasma lipid levels and the interactions between food components can be quite complex. The major break-through for dietary treatment of high cholesterol levels came in the early 1950s when Kinsell and co-workers showed that when saturated fats were replaced isocalorically by fat rich in polyunsaturated fat, serum cholesterol falls. This now well-documented fact, the corner stone of dietary lipid management, is well known not only by the medical profession but also by the general public.

A major aim of the dietary advice is directed towards reduction of LDL-C, the concentration of which is reflected by the level of total-C. In general these diets are recommended to have a total fat intake that is 30% or less of total energy intake with a content of saturated fat 10% or less of the energy intake, a dietary cholesterol intake <300 mg/day (for example an ordinary egg typically contains about 250 mg of cholesterol) and a replacement of saturated fat by mono/polyunsaturated fat. ATP III stressed the need for TLC to include recommendations of a reduced intake of saturated fats as well as of cholesterol in the diet. Their recommendations are shown in detail in Figure 10.1.

Exercise and lipid management

A sedentary life style is associated with an increased risk of CVD and obesity; the beneficial effects of exercise, at work or in leisure time, on prevention of CHD have been shown in several epidemiological studies. However, in spite of these clinical and epidemiological observations, well-controlled studies on the effects of exercise on blood lipids are sparse. It is relatively well established that extreme cohorts of intensive marathon runners in addition to be lean have low levels of atherogenic

Therapeutic lifestyle changes diet: nutrient composition of the TLC diet	
Nutrient	**Recommended intake**
Saturated fat*	<7% of total calories
Polyunsaturated fat	≤10% of total calories
Monounsaturated fat	≤20% of total calories
Total fat	25–30% of total calories
Carbohydrate†	50–60% of total calories
Fibre	20–30 g/day
Protein	Approximately 15% of total calories
Cholesterol	<200 mg/day
Total calories‡	Balance energy intake and expenditure to maintain desirable body weight/prevent weight gain

Figure 10.1 Therapeutic lifestyle changes diet: nutrient composition of the TLC diet. *Trans fatty acids are another low-density lipoprotein raising fat that should be kept at a low intake. †Carbohydrates should be derived predominantly from foods rich in complex carbohydrates including grains, especially whole grains, fruits and vegetables. ‡Daily energy expenditure should include at least moderate physical activity (contributing approximately 200 kcal/day). Reproduced with permission from ATP III. JAMA 2001;285:2486-2497.

plasma lipids but high levels of protective HDL. In general recommendations on exercise training include aerobic exercise such as brisk walking, jogging, swimming and biking for at least an 30 minutes a day, 5 days a week or more.

The effects of exercise training on blood lipids can be summarised as follows:

- total-C and LDL-C: little or no effect
- triglycerides: decrease
- HDL-C: increase, but variable

To sum up, the effects of exercise training on the lipid profile are modest. However, it should not be forgotten that exercise can have other metabolic effects that may be beneficial in the prevention of risk for CVDs and diabetes such as enhancing insulin sensitivity (i.e. reducing insulin resistance) and glycaemic control and also for the quality of life

Pharmacotherapy

If the lipid levels have not been normalised or the goals for lipid levels specifically defined for a given patient have not been reached by life style changes and other means such as glycaemic control in diabetes, then pharmacological lipid-modifying treatment has to be considered while continuing the life style recommendations.

Classes of lipid-modifying drugs

The complete pharmacological collection of lipid-modifying drugs includes a number of different drugs with diverse effects on the lipid profile and various modes of action. The main classes of lipid-modifying drugs presently in use are:

- statins
- nicotinic acid (niacin)
- fibrates
- bile acid sequestrants (resins)
- cholesterol absorption inhibitors

These drugs can be used either in monotherapy or in combination. For patients with severe hyperlipidaemia, often with a genetic cause such as FH, a combination of drugs may need to be used to achieve a satisfactory outcome. If statins are tolerated the most usual combination therapy is a statin plus a drug from the other classes of lipid-modifying drugs, e.g. nicotinic acid or cholesterol absorption inhibitors.

How to chose a lipid-modifying drug

The choice of a lipid-modifying drug depends on many factors. As a start for the selection of a lipid-modifying drug based on the type of the patient's dyslipidaemia a simple 'rule of the thumb' is given in Figure 10.2.

Overview of the properties of the classes of lipid-modifying drugs

An overview of properties of the different classes of lipid-modifying drugs in clinical use is given in Figure 10.3 which shows the main lipoprotein/lipid effects, adverse effects, contraindications and a summary of clinical results.

Rule of thumb for choice of lipid-modifying drugs			
Type of dyslipidaemia	Fredrickson/ WHO classification	First choice	Second choice*
High LDL (hypercholesterolaemia)	IIA	Statin	Ezetimibe
			Resins
			Nicotinic acid
High LDL + high VLDL (combined hyperlipidaemia)	IIB	Statin	Fibrate (other than gemfibrozil)
			Ezetimibe
			Nicotinic acid
High VLDL (hypertriglceridaemia)	IV	Fibrate	Statin
			Nicotinic acid
High VLDL + chylomicronaemia	V	Nicotinic acid	Fibrate
			Omega 3
Low HDL	–	Nicotinic acid	Fibrate

Figure 10.2 Rule of thumb for choice of lipid-modifying drugs. *Given either as monotherapy when the first choice is not tolerated or in combination with the first choice to obtain a better effect.

Overview of lipid-lowering drugs in clinical use

Lipid or lipoprotein effect (%)*	Adverse effects	Contraindications	Clinical trial results
Drug class: Statins (HMG-CoA reductase inhibitors)			
LDL ↓ 18–55 HDL ↑ 5–15 TG ↓ 7–30	Myopathy Increased liver enzymes	Absolute: • Active or chronic liver disease Relative: • Concomitant use of certain drugs‡	Reduced major coronary events, CHD deaths, need for coronary procedures, stroke and total mortality
Drug class: Nicotinic acid†			
LDL ↓ 5–25 HDL ↑ 15–35 TG ↓ 20–50	Flushing Hyperglycaemia Hyperuricaemia (or gout) Upper gastrointestinal distress Hepatotoxicity	Absolute: • Chronic liver disease • Severe gout Relative: • Hyperuricaemia • Peptic ulcer disease	Reduced major coronary events, and possibly total mortality
Drug class: Fibrates (fibric acids)			
LDL ↓ 5–25 (may be increased in patients with high TG) HDL ↑ 10–20 TG ↓ 20–50	Dyspepsia Gallstones Myopathy	Absolute: • Severe renal disease • Severe hepatic disease	Reduced major coronary events
Drug class: cholesterol absorption inhibitors			
LDL ↓ 10–20 HDL ↑ 0–5 TG ↓ 0–5	Dyspepsia Constipation Diarrhoea Myopathy	Absolute: • Gastrointestinal disease • Liver disease	No clinical end point studies available, best results in combination with statins and fibrates
Drug class: Resins (bile acid sequestrants)			
LDL ↓ 15–30 HDL ↑ 3–5 TG, no change or increase	Gastrointestinal distress Constipation Decreased absorption of other drugs	Absolute: • Dysbetalipo-proteinaemia • TG >10.3 mmol/L Relative: • TG >5.2 mmol/L	Reduced major coronary events and CHD deaths

Figure 10.3 Overview of lipid-lowering drugs in clinical use. *Dose dependent, particularly for statins, resins and nicotinic acid; †In severe type V hyperlipidaemia (triglycerides 50–100 mmol/L) with frequent attacks of pancreatitis, plain nicotinic acid 12–15 g/day has been used, resulting in complete freedom from attacks (it is remarkably well tolerated for many years; Carlson LA, personal experience). ‡Cyclosporine, macrolide antibiotics, various antifungal agents and cytochrome P450 inhibitors (fibrates and nicotinic acid should be used with appropriate caution). Adapted with permission from Expert Panel on Detection, Evaluation, and Treatment of High Blood Cholesterol in Adults. JAMA 2001; 285:2486–2497. ©2001 American Medical Association.

Chapter 11

Drugs for lipid management

Statins

The discovery of statins and the early ground-breaking clinical results with statins are described above in Chapter 8. The efficacy of statins to reduce new events of clinical atherosclerosis in primary as well as secondary prevention is evident from an extensive almost overwhelming literature on the subject. There is no doubt that patients at risk for clinical atherosclerosis, irrespective of lipid risk factors, will benefit from statins as first-line treatment, however, it may well have to be combined with other. Lipid management drugs depending on the type of dyslipidaemia and the response to statins. It is worth noting that there is a residual risk after treatment with statins of clinical atherosclerosis events that varies between 40–60%.

Dose-response: LDL-C

There are six marketed statins in current use which are listed in Figure 11.1 with their recommended starting doses, maximum doses and LDL-C lowering effects. It can be seen in this list that the degree of LDL-C lowering varies between the available statins and that there is a dose-response effect on LDL-C especially for the four doses of both atorvastatin and rosuvastatin, the maximum dose the decrease of LDL-C was about 60% with atorvastatin and rosuvastatin.

The dose response effect on the changes in LDL-C and HDL-C induced by rosuvastatin, atorvastatin, simvastatin and pravastatin was studied in the STELLAR trial [50], a randomised, open-label comparator-controlled study comprising 2431 hypercholesterolaemic patients. The results of

STELLAR are shown in Figure 11.2 and Figure 11.3 for LDL-C and HDL-C, respectively. For LDL-C there was a linear decrease with increasing doses of the four statins, most pronounced with rosuvastatin and atorvastatin (Figure 11.2). After 6 weeks' treatment rosuvastatin had reduced LDL-C 8% more than atorvastatin, 12–18% more than simvastatin and 26% more than pravastatin.

The LDL-C goals of ATP III were achieved by 82–89% of the patients in the rosuvastatin groups (dose 10–40 mg/day) and by 69–85% of subjects treated with atorvastatin (dose 10–80 mg/day). The European LDL-C goal of <3.0 mmol/L (116 mg/dL) was reached by 79–92% and 52–81% in the rosuvastatin and atorvastatin groups, respectively.

Rosuvastatin, simvastatin and pravastatin raised HDL-C 2–10% (Figure 11.3). Rosuvastatin 40 mg had the most effect on HDL-C while atorvastatin 80 mg had the least effect. In summary the STELLAR trial as well as several other trials have clearly demonstrated that rosuvastatin is the most potent marketed LDL-lowering statin with atorvastatin coming in as the second most potent.

LDL cholesterol-lowering efficacy of starting and maximum doses of statins				
	Starting dose		Maximum dose	
Statin	Dose (mg)	Average LDL-C reduction (%)	Dose (mg)	Average LDL-C reduction (%)
Atorvastatin	10	39	80	60
	20	43		
	40*	50		
Fluvastatin	40	25	80 XL	35
	40 b.i.d	36		
	80 XL	35		
Lovastatin	20	27	40 b.i.d.	40
Pravastatin	40	34	80	37
Rosuvastatin	5	45	40	63
	10	52		
	20†	55		
Simvastatin	20	38	80	47
	40	41		

Figure 11.1 LDL cholesterol-lowering efficacy of starting and maximum doses of statins.
*40 mg starting dose can be used when need LDL-C reduction >45%. †20 mg starting dose can be used when aggressive lipid target required for marked hypercholesterolaemia (LDL-C >4.9 mmol/L, >190 mg/dL). C, cholesterol; LDL, low-density lipoprotein; XL, extended-release. Adapted from [43].

STELLAR trial: percentage change from baseline levels of LDL-C

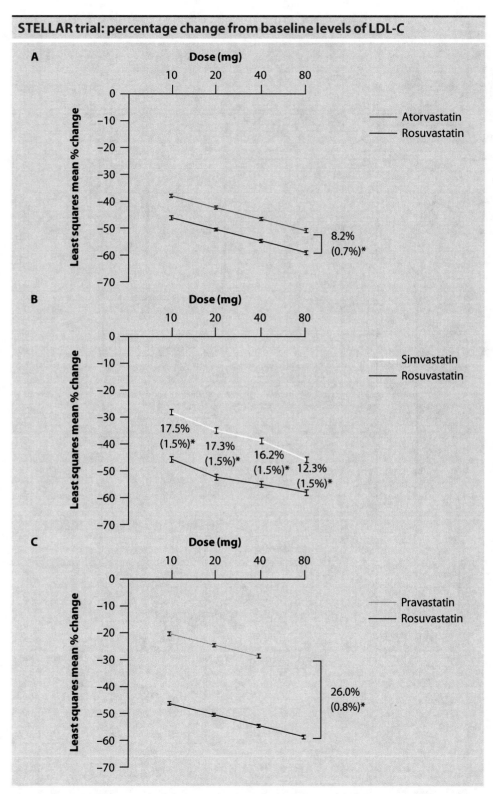

Figure 11.2 STELLAR trial: percentage change from baseline levels of LDL-C. Changes at week 6 across dose ranges are shown (difference across dose range for rosuvastatin vs simvastatin could not be calculated, because the slopes were nonparallel). *p <0.001. HDL-C, high-density lipoprotein cholesterol. Data from [50].

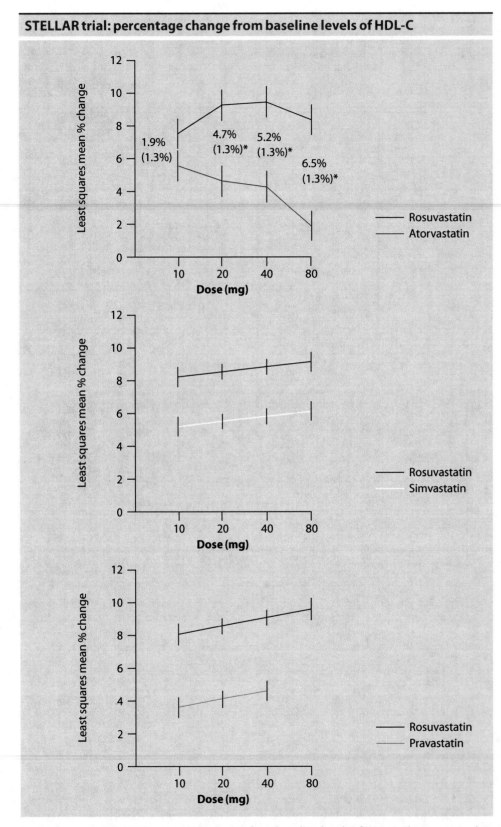

Figure 11.3 STELLAR trial: percentage change from baseline levels of HDL-C. Changes at week 6 across dose ranges are shown. *p <0.001. HDL-C, high-density lipoprotein cholesterol. Data from [50].

Adverse effects

The statins in current use have remarkably few side effects, drug tolerance was similar for all statins in the STELLAR trial. Increases of aminotransferases may occur in approximately 5% of statin treated patients and elevations are transient. Myalgia with or without increase in creatinine kinase (CK) is a rare side-effect which requires careful follow-up because of the risk of rhabdomyolysis which has been reported to occur with an incidence rate of 0.6–1.6/10,000 person years in patients treated with statins currently in use. One statin, the extremely potent cerivastatin, has been withdrawn from the market due to a high incidence rate of rhabdomyolysis.

Pleiotropic, cholesterol-independent effects

As for many other lipid-modifying drugs, statins have been shown to have a number of other effects than reducing plasma cholesterol levels, so called pleiotropic effects, which might contribute to their beneficial effects on clinical atherosclerosis although this has so far not been proven. Among these effects are improvement of endothelial function occurring before cholesterol is lowered and attenuation of inflammatory processes which is associated with a decrease of the inflammatory marker and CHD risk factor CRP. Of unknown clinical importance is the inhibitory effect of statins on the Rho/Rho kinase which appear to be involved in experimental atherosclerosis.

Summary of effects of nicotinic acid on plasma lipoprotein classes

Lipoprotein	Effect
Chylomicrons	
VLDL	↓
Beta-VLDL	↓
IDL	↓
LDL	↓
Small, dense LDL	↓
HDL	↑
HDL$_2$	↑
Lp(a)	↓

Figure 11.4 Summary of effects of nicotinic acid on plasma lipoprotein classes. HDL, high-density lipoprotein; IDL, intermediate-density lipoprotein; LDL, low-density lipoprotein; Lp(a), lipoprotein (a); VLDL, very low-density lipoprotein.

Nicotinic acid (niacin)

The cholesterol-lowering effect of nicotinic acid was discovered approximately 50 years ago by the Canadian pathologist Altschul. The early discovered lipid effects of nicotinic acid, as well as those currently known, which involve all major lipoprotein classes – the apoB-containing lipoproteins, from chylomicrons via VLDL and LDL to Lp(a) and the apoA-containing HDL lipoproteins are summarised in Figure 11.4 and have recently been reviewed [51]. This review also describes the early clinical and metabolic studies with this drug and the early trials showing the beneficial effects of treatment with nicotinic acid either as monotherapy or in combination with other lipid-modifying drugs, such as fibrates and above all statins, on outcomes of clinical atherosclerosis, in particular two ground-breaking trials the Coronary Drug Project (CDP) [52] and HATS [53]. Different preparations of nicotinic acid for clinical use are described below.

Prevention of clinical atherosclerosis

CDP was a secondary prevention placebo-controlled trial [52], conducted between 1966 to 1974 in 53 clinical centres in the USA. The patients were treated with immediate-release nicotinic acid (IRN), 3 g/day for 6.5 years which resulted in significant reductions of several manifestations of clinical atherosclerosis, including myocardial infarctions, stroke and angina compared to placebo as shown in Figure 11.5. In the long-term follow up of CDP (15 years) mortality had decreased by 11% for those given nicotinic acid.

The Stockholm Ischaemic Heart Disease Secondary Prevention Study randomised consecutive survivors of myocardial infarction in one Stockholm hospital 1972–1976 to either a treatment group given the combination of IRN 3 g plus clofibrate 2 g daily at discharge after the acute episode for five years (n=276) or one control group receiving ordinary treatment (n=279) [56]. Total cholesterol and triglycerides were reduced by 13% and 19%, respectively, compared to controls. Total mortality (Figure 11.6) and IHD mortality were reduced by 26% and 36%, respectively.

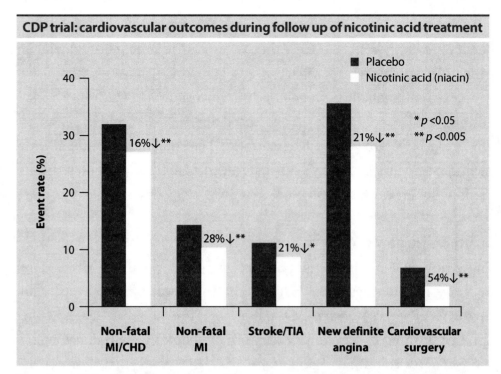

Figure 11.5 CDP trial: cardiovascular outcomes during follow up of nicotinic acid treatment. Clinical cardiovascular outcomes were reduced significantly, the predefined primary event (total mortality) being reduced by 4.3% (n.s.). CHD, coronary heart disease; MI, myocardial infarction; TIA, transient ischaemic attack. Adapted from [54].

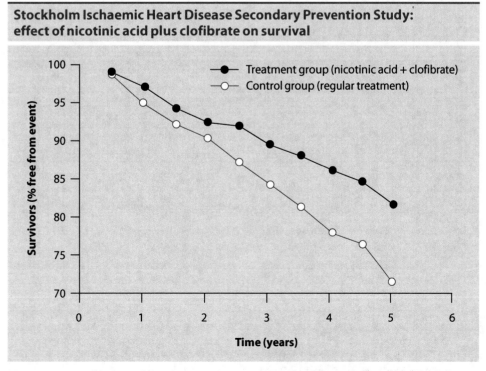

Figure 11.6 Stockholm Ischaemic Heart Disease Secondary Prevention Study: effect of nicotinic acid plus clofibrate on survival. Intention to treat principle. Data from [55].

A recent review [53] has summarised the clinical results of the secondary prevention HATS (HDL Atherosclerosis Treatment Study) trial in which 160 patients with coronary disease and low HDL were randomised to active treatment with extended-release nicotinic acid (ERN) with simvastatin or placebo. LDL-C was decreased and HDL-C raised by 42% and 26%, respectively, by the active treatment. The combined treatment with nicotinic acid (Niaspan) and simvastatin compared to placebo reduced cardiovascular events by 60–90% (Figure 11.7).

Lipid management

The treatment of dyslipidaemic patients with 4 g/day of IRN (in use before ERN preparations became available) and the resulting broad spectrum lipid effects of this treatment is shown in Figure 11.8. The levels of the apoB-containing lipoproteins VLDL, LDL and Lp(a) were reduced while those of apoA-containing lipoproteins HDL, HDL_3 and particularly HDL_2 were increased.

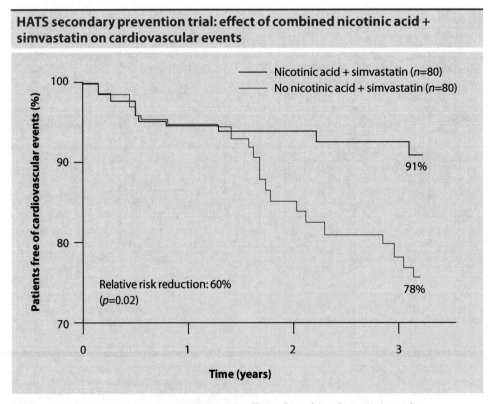

Figure 11.7 HATS secondary prevention trial: effect of combined nicotinic acid + simvastatin on cardiovascular events. Data from [56].

Dose-response: lipoproteins

For all lipoprotein classes there is a dose-response effect of nicotinic acid as shown in Figure 11.9 with doses of ERN ranging from 30 to 3000 mg/day for LDL-C, HDL-C, Lp(a) and plasma triglycerides. It is worth noting that:

- the dose-response is equally pronounced for the HDL-C raising effect as for the lowering of the apoB;
- the dose-containing lipoproteins in one and the same patient cohort, suggesting a common mode of action;
- when treated with 3000 mg of nicotinic acid HDL-C increased by 29% and LDL-C, Lp(a) and triglycerides decreased by 21%, 26% and 44%, respectively.

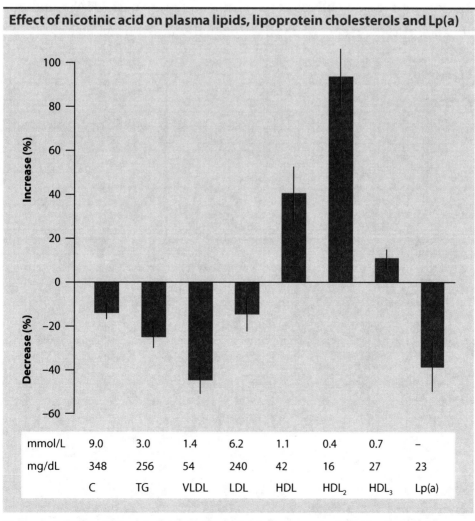

Figure 11.8 Effect of nicotinic acid on plasma lipids, lipoprotein cholesterols and Lp(a).
Mean ± SEM for 31 dyslipidaemic subjects treated with 4 g of nicotinic acid daily for 6 weeks.
C, cholesterol; HDL, high-density lipoprotein; LDL, low-density lipoprotein; Lp(a), lipoprotein (a);
TG, triglycerides; VLDL, very low-density lipoprotein. Data from [57].

Effect of combining nicotinic acid with other lipid-modifying drugs

An attractive combination therapy is with a LDL-lowering drug like statins and the HDL-raising nicotinic acid, which was used in the HATS trial. A compilation of the effect of treatment with the combination of varying doses of nicotinic acid (Niaspan) and a statin (lovastatin) on the lipid profile is given in Figure 11.10. Using this combination of the two lipid-modifying drugs at the highest doses LDL-C was reduced by as much as 45% and HDL-C was increased by 41%.

Lipid management by combination of nicotinic acid with other lipid-modifying drugs has resulted in improved lipid effects when compared to the use of single drugs. The beneficial clinical outcomes for the combination of nicotinic acid with either a statin or a fibrate in the HATS and the Stockholm study, respectively, have been discussed previously.

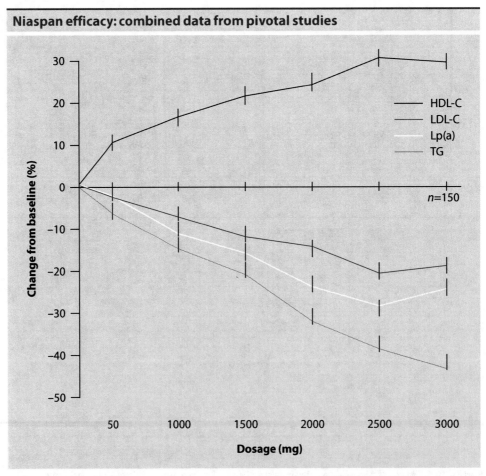

Figure 11.9 Niaspan efficacy: combined data from pivotal studies. HDL-C, high-density lipoprotein cholesterol; LDL-C, low-density lipoprotein cholesterol; Lp(a), lipoprotein (a); TG, triglycerides. Adapted from [58].

Flushing on nicotinic acid administration

Flushing is a pathognomonic, inevitable but harmless adverse effect of treatment with nicotinic acid. It starts in the face and the higher the dose the more rapidly it spreads over the upper part of the body. The duration is around one hour after 1 g of IRN.

The flush has been shown to be caused by a release of prostaglandin D2 (PGD$_2$) from dermal Langerhans cells which are activated when nicotinic acid is bound to the Gi-coupled newly discovered nicotinic acid receptor (HM74). When PGD$_2$ is bound to its receptor D1P vasodilation and thus flush is initiated. Recently a PGD$_2$ receptor antagonist compound, laropiprant, has been found to inhibit nicotinic acid induced flush without modifying the lipid effects of this drug [60,61].

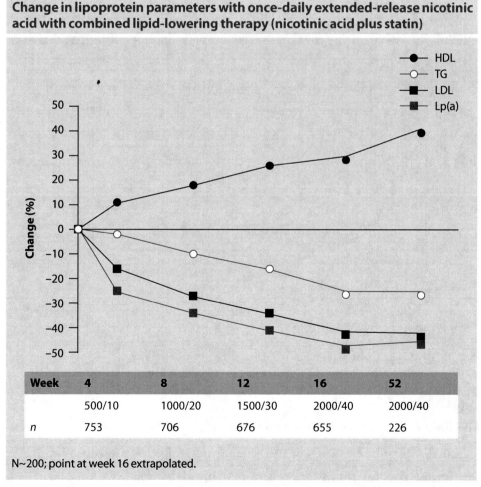

Change in lipoprotein parameters with once-daily extended-release nicotinic acid with combined lipid-lowering therapy (nicotinic acid plus statin)

Week	4	8	12	16	52
	500/10	1000/20	1500/30	2000/40	2000/40
n	753	706	676	655	226

N~200; point at week 16 extrapolated.

Figure 11.10 Change in lipoprotein parameters with once-daily extended-release nicotinic acid with combined lipid-lowering therapy (nicotinic acid plus statin). HDL, high-density lipoprotein; LDL, low-density lipoprotein; Lp(a), lipoprotein (a); TG, triglycerides. Data from [59].

Current nicotinic acid drugs

Nicotinic acid as a lipid-modifying drug was from the beginning used as plain (crystalline) nicotinic acid and IRN. The side effects, particularly those of the immediate flushing has limited the use of IRN in lipid management. Sustained-release (SR) formulations were developed in the hope of diminishing the flush, however, the SR preparations were associated with hepatotoxicity and have been abandoned in clinical use. An ERN preparation (Niaspan) with absorption rates between IR and SR preparations has been developed and has now been in use for several years [62]. ERN preparation (Niaspan) taken once daily at bedtime gives rise to much less flush than IRN, but some flushing still occurs with ERN. It has, however, identical lipid-modifying properties as IRN.

The latest advancement for nicotinic acid in lipid management is the combination of Niaspan with laropiprant (for specific inhibition of the flush) which is available on the market as Tredaptive. A cohort of more than 400 dyslipidaemic patients were randomised to placebo, Niaspan 1 g or the combination of Niaspan 1 g with laropiprant for several weeks treatment [60]. The flush, particularly severe and extreme manifestations, were significantly reduced by this combination laropiprant as shown in Figure 11.11. The nicotinic acid effects on HDL-C, LDL-C and triglycerides were not modified by the addition of laropiprant to nicotinic acid (Figure 11.12).

Presently there are four types of nicotinic acid preparations available in 1 g (or lower) doses for clinical use in lipid management:
- IRN (crystalline-nicotinic acid),
- ERN (Niaspan),
- fixed-dose combinations of ERN and statins (Advicor, Simcor) are available in the USA, and
- combination of ERN and laropiprant (Tredaptive)

Fibrates

The lipid effects of clofibrate, the first fibrate, were discovered and published 1962 [63] and brought into the clinic and published in 1963 [64]. Clofibrate was for many years the leading drug for lowering lipids in clinical practice, but second generation fibrates (gemfibrozil, fenofibrate, bezafibrate and ciprofibrate) were soon to appear on the market.

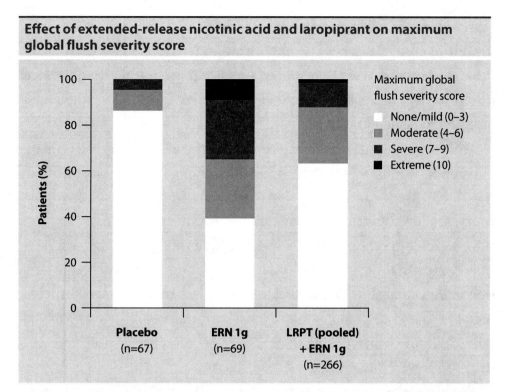

Figure 11.11 Effect of extended-release nicotinic acid and laropiprant on maximum global flush severity score. ERN, extended-release nicotinic acid; LRPT, laropiprant. Data from [60].

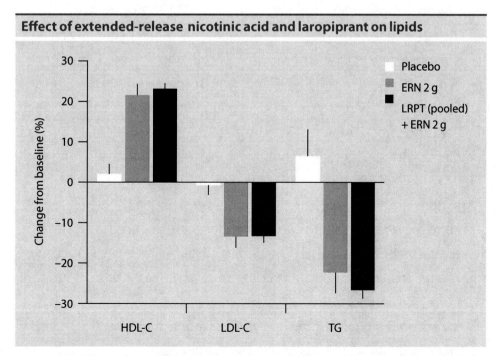

Figure 11.12 Effect of extended-release nicotinic acid and laropiprant on lipids. The mean percentage change from baseline at week 8 is shown (with standard error). LRPT, laropiprant; C, cholesterol; HDL, high-density lipoprotein; LDL, low-density lipoprotein; TG, triglycerides. Data from [60].

Prevention of clinical atherosclerosis

Results of trials studying clinical outcomes of treatment with fibrates have given different results over the years leading to the questions 'Which fibrate, which patients, what mechanisms? [65], a further important question to be added is 'What clinical results?'.

The first large trial using monotherapy with clofibrate was the primary prevention WHO/clofibrate trial in which hypercholesterolaemic men (n=10,000)were randomised for placebo or clofibrate treatment for five years [66]. Pretreatment mean cholesterol level was 6.42 mmol/L (247 mg/dL), the cholesterol decrease in clofibrate treated men was 9%. There was a significant 25% reduction in non-fatal myocardial infarction but no change in CHD mortality. However, there was a significant increase in non-CHD mortality of unspecific nature in the men treated with clofibrate which of course limited the acceptance of clofibrate as a drug for prevention of clinical atherosclerosis.

However, the good effects of fibrates on VLDL and HDL lead to further clinical trials. Two of the earliest trials to examine the new fibrate gemfibrozil were the Helsinki Heart Study (HHS) [67] and the Veterans Affairs High-Density Lipoprotein Intervention Trial (VA-HIT) [68].

The HHS was a primary prevention placebo-controlled study treated dyslipidaemic men with the fibrate gemfibrozil for 5 years. Triglycerides and LDL-C were reduced by 35% and 11%, respectively, HDL increased by 11%. Importantly there was a 34% reduction in CHD events although there was no effect on mortality; the clinical effects were most evident in patients with the metabolic syndrome. VA-HIT randomised men with CHD and low HDL for treatment with gemfibrozil or placebo for five years, approximately half of the patients in this trial had metabolic syndrome or type 2 diabetes. Triglycerides were reduced by 31%, LDL remained unchanged and HDL rose by 7.7%. Major events of clinical atherosclerosis were reduced by 22% and there was a non-significant reduction of total mortality.

The lipid effects of fibrates are indeed tailored for the treatment of diabetic dyslipidaemia as discussed in Chapter 12.

Summary of clinical outcomes of fibrate trials

The effects of fibrates on outcomes of clinical atherosclerosis have recently been summarised in a systematic review and meta-analysis by Jun et al. [69], the condensed the results of 18 trials comprising data from 45,000 participants including 2870 major cardiovascular events and 3880 deaths.

Overall fibrate therapy reduced the risk of coronary events by 13% as shown in Figure 11.13 which also details the individual results of 16 of the trials. The review clearly shows that the degree of clinical benefit was related to the level of triglycerides. Furthermore treatment with fibrates was most beneficial the lower the triglyceride levels. The conclusion of this review was that fibrate therapy reduces the risk of CVD by preventing coronary events and that as modern fibrates are safe and well-tolerated these agents have a role in cardiac protection.

Lipid management

The main lipid effect of fibrates is to decrease the levels of VLDL resulting in a reduction of triglycerides, and to raise HDL, resulting in an increase of HDL-C. Treatment with fibrates only slightly reduces the concentration of LDL-C. A recent detailed analysis of lipoprotein subclasses by NMR spectroscopy in the VA-HIT trial showed that gemfibrozil increased the size of LDL particles and lowered the number of LDL particles while raising the number of HDL particles and small HDL subclass particles [83]. The particle concentrations of LDL and HDL were independently predictive of new CHD events in this trial, LDL positively and HDL negatively. However, the particle size of LDL and HDL were not related to the clinical outcomes.

On the molecular level fibrates exert their effects on the lipid profile by activation of the peroxisome proliferator activated receptor (PPAR), a transcription factor controlling genes associated with lipoprotein metabolism causing increased expression of, for example, lipoprotein lipase, reverse cholesterol transport factors (ABCA1) and HDL apolipoproteins such as apoA-I.

Effect of fibrates on the risk of coronary events

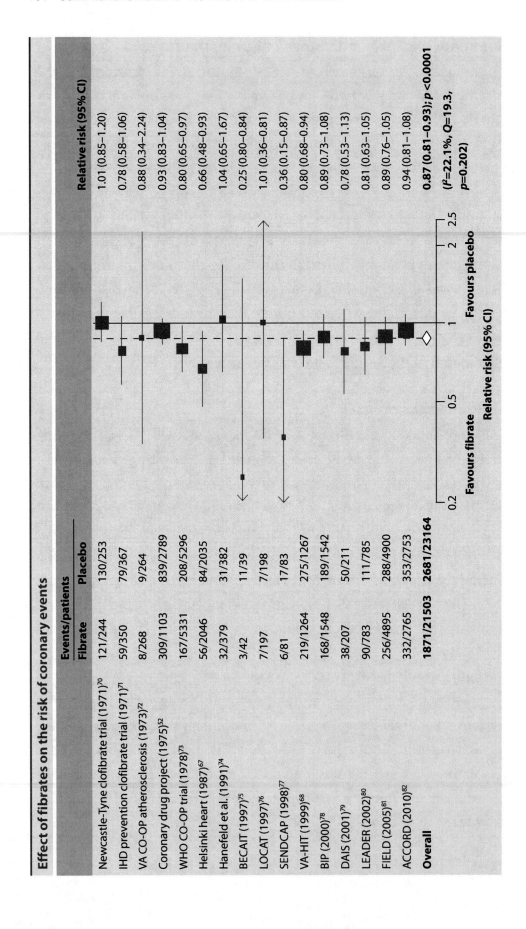

	Events/patients		Relative risk (95% CI)
	Fibrate	Placebo	
Newcastle-Tyne clofibrate trial (1971)[70]	121/244	130/253	1.01 (0.85–1.20)
IHD prevention clofibrate trial (1971)[71]	59/350	79/367	0.78 (0.58–1.06)
VA CO-OP atherosclerosis (1973)[72]	8/268	9/264	0.88 (0.34–2.24)
Coronary drug project (1975)[52]	309/1103	839/2789	0.93 (0.83–1.04)
WHO CO-OP trial (1978)[73]	167/5331	208/5296	0.80 (0.65–0.97)
Helsinki heart (1987)[67]	56/2046	84/2035	0.66 (0.48–0.93)
Hanefeld et al. (1991)[74]	32/379	31/382	1.04 (0.65–1.67)
BECAIT (1997)[75]	3/42	11/39	0.25 (0.80–0.84)
LOCAT (1997)[76]	7/197	7/198	1.01 (0.36–0.81)
SENDCAP (1998)[77]	6/81	17/83	0.36 (0.15–0.87)
VA-HIT (1999)[68]	219/1264	275/1267	0.80 (0.68–0.94)
BIP (2000)[78]	168/1548	189/1542	0.89 (0.73–1.08)
DAIS (2001)[79]	38/207	50/211	0.78 (0.53–1.13)
LEADER (2002)[80]	90/783	111/785	0.81 (0.63–1.05)
FIELD (2005)[81]	256/4895	288/4900	0.89 (0.76–1.05)
ACCORD (2010)[82]	332/2765	353/2753	0.94 (0.81–1.08)
Overall	**1871/21503**	**2681/23164**	**0.87 (0.81–0.93); p <0.0001**
			(I^2=22.1%, Q=19.3, p=0.202)

(See opposite) Figure 11.13 Effect of fibrates on the risk of coronary events. Reproduced with permission from [69].

Current fibrate drugs

The available fibrate drugs and their recommended daily standard doses in common clinical practice are:

- fenofibrate – 200 mg
- gemfibrozil – 1200 mg (600 mg twice daily)
- bezafibrate – 400 mg
- ciprofibrate – 100 mg

Bile acid sequestrants (resins)

Cholesterol is synthesised in the liver and can only be broken down in this organ to become bile acids which are secreted into the intestines. This is one of the metabolic pathways for the elimination cholesterol from the body. The bile acids after secretion into the intestines are normally reabsorbed to over 95%. The bile acid sequestrants (BAS) work by binding bile acids in the gut and therefore inhibit their reabsorption, leading to bile acid excretion from the body via faeces. In this way the elimination of cholesterol from the body is enhanced, the hepatic cholesterol pool diminished and the increased demand for cholesterol in the liver leads to an upregulation of the hepatic LDL receptors with an increased uptake of cholesterol rich LDL from the blood leading to reduced levels of LDL.

The first BAS (cholestyramine), an anion exchange resin and a large molecule, it is neither digested nor absorbed; cholestyramine appeared in the 1950s and is still in use, it is supplied as a powder which has to be dispersed in liquid. It was shown to lower plasma cholesterol in a dose-dependent way with 20% or more in doses of 24 g/day divided into two or three daily doses. It was demonstrated in the early stages of the CDPP trial that the lowering of cholesterol by high doses of cholestyramine exerted beneficial effects on the occurrence of clinical atherosclerosis, see Chapter 8. The major side-effect is obstipation, sometimes severe. In the seven-year CDPP trial one third of the patients stopped taking cholestyramine due to adverse effects, mainly obstipation.

Colestipol and colesevelam are two more recently developed BAS in clinical use. Colesevelam appears to cause less problem with constipation than the earlier non-selective BAS but be effective as a cholesterol-reducing drug. BAS have been shown to be effective cholesterol-lowering drugs with beneficial effects on clinical atherosclerosis and are without direct systemic effects, however as they are not absorbed their use as monotherapy today is quite limited, in part due to the high dosage levels, constipation and possible interference with the absorption of other drugs and certain nutrients. They can, however, have a possible role added on to other lipid-modifying drugs in the treatment of severe hypercholesterolaemia as in cases of pronounced FH.

Cholesterol absorption inhibitors
Intestinal cholesterol balance, lipid management and ezetimibe

Ever since the ground-breaking animal experiments of the Russian pathologist Anitschkow in the beginning of the 20th century, whose studies showed that dietary cholesterol fed to rabbits caused atherosclerosis, the role of dietary cholesterol has now and then had a central place in the discussions on the pathogenesis of clinical atherosclerosis and its treatment. ATP III recommends a dietary intake of <200 mg/day in the recommendations of the TLC diet (see Figure 10.1). Approximately 1200 mg of cholesterol per day will enter the gut, 300 mg from the diet and 900 mg via the bile from the liver. Of this cholesterol load 600 mg is normally reabsorbed into the liver and 600 mg excreted via the faeces.

Ezetimibe is a recently developed specific inhibitor of intestinal cholesterol reabsorption, acting at the intestinal brush border by inhibiting the cholesterol transport protein Niemann-Pick C1-like 1 protein. Ezetimibe diminishes the reabsorption of cholesterol to approximately 300 mg leading to an increased faecal excretion of cholesterol of about 900 mg/day. The ensuing reduced inflow of cholesterol back to the hepatic cholesterol pool causes a compensatory stimulation of hepatic LDL receptor activity which leads to increased hepatic uptake of the cholesterol-rich LDL from the blood, hence the LDL level will decrease while the liver is supplied with cholesterol. Ezetimibe given once daily in a dose of 10 mg reduces plasma levels of LDL-C by approximately 20%. However, this drug is more often used in combination therapy, mostly with statins, than in monotherapy. The combination of ezetimibe with statins has an excellent effect on LDL-C. In a trial conducted in 34 UK primary care centres with 1748 patients at high-risk for clinical athero-sclerosis and LDL-C >2.0 mmol/L (77 mg/dL), the goal recommended by the Joint British Societies (see Chapter 9), were randomised to three treatment groups:

• ezetimibe/simvastatin 10/40 mg,

• atorvastatin 40 mg, or

• rosuvastatin 5-10 mg.

Average pre-treatment LDL-C was 2.6 mmol/L (101 mg/dL). The primary outcome measure was the proportion of patients reaching the LDL-C goal of 2.0 mmol/L (77 mg/dL) [84]. Figure 11.14 shows the effect of the three treatments on LDL-C, the combination therapy with ezetimibe and simvastatin was clearly superior for both LDL-C and total-C compared to the other two treatments.

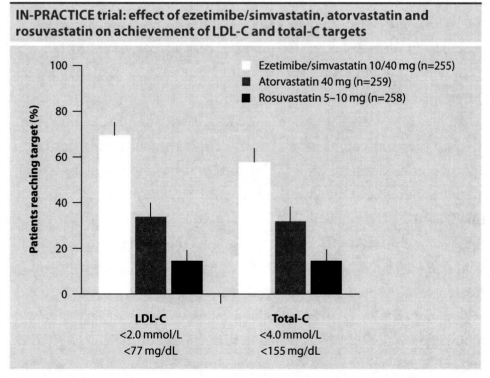

Figure 11.14 IN-PRACTICE trial: effect of ezetimibe/simvastatin, atorvastatin and rosuvastatin on achievement of low-density lipoprotein cholesterol (LDL-C) and total cholesterol (C) targets. Data from [84].

Effect of the combination of ezetimibe with a statin on carotid intima-media thickness

Three recent trials (ENHANCE, SANDS, ARBITER) have assessed what effect the addition of ezetimibe to statin treatment in high-risk patients on carotid intima-media thickness (CIMT), a commonly used risk surrogate measure for atherosclerosis, in the latter trial moreover compared to the effect of also addition of niacin. In the ENHANCE trial, patients with FH, n=720 and LDL-C >5.4 mmol/L (210 mg/dL) were randomised for treatment with 80 mg of simvastatin with either placebo or ezetimibe 10 mg for two years [85]. After two years' treatment LDL-C concentration was 5.0 mmol/L (193 mg/dL) and 3.7 mmol/L (141 mg/dL) in the simvastatin/placebo group and the simvastatin/ezetimibe group, respectively (p <0.01 for this 16.5% difference).

The primary outcome was the mean change in CIMT which did not differ significantly between the two groups in spite of the much lower LDL levels achieved in the ezetimibe group. Of note is that the combined treatment also reduced CRP 26% more than statin treatment alone.

The unexpected results of ENHANCE have raised much discussion about the clinical utility of ezetimibe. A careful analysis of ENHANCE by Brown and Taylor [86] have suggested four possible explanations for the unforeseen negative clinical outcomes. Of these suggestions, the possibility that pre-treatment of FH patients with statins, before entering into the trial, might have altered the plaques with lipid depletion and so rendered them less sensitive to LDL lowering, is a plausible but unproven hypothesis. Furthermore, the American College of Cardiology (ACC) issued a recommendation soon after the publication of ENHANCE that 'major clinical decisions not be made on the basis of the ENHANCE study' [87]. The judicious comment of Brown and Taylor concerning treatment of dyslipidaemic patients was: '*First, achieve targets for levels of LDL and HDL cholesterol with the use of statins plus drugs that have shown clinical benefits when added to statins (e.g. nicotinic acid, fibrates and bile acid sequestrants), as tolerated. Second, use ezetimibe in patients who, despite the above-mentioned therapy do not achieve their individual targets. And third, wait for clarifying studies.*'

The Stop Atherosclerosis in Native Diabetics Study (SANDS) comprised 499 American Indian men (a population with high prevalence of diabetes) randomised to:

- standard treatment goals – LDL-C 2.6 mmol/L (100 mg/dL), non-HDL-C 3.4 mmol/L (130 mg/dL), SBP 130 mmHg, and
- aggressive treatment goals – 1.8 mmol/L (70 mg/dL), 2.6 mmol/L (100 mg/dL) and 115 mmHg [88].

Both schedules followed the recommendations of ATP III starting with TLC. If LDL-C goals were not met by TLC a statin was added. If the LDL-C was not reached with a statin alone ezetimibe was added. The standard treatment group comprised 204 patients, the aggressive treatment group 223 subjects (154 on statin alone, 69 on statin plus ezetimibe). During the 36 months of follow-up no significant changes occurred in BMI or HbA1c. The effect on CIMT is illustrated for the three groups in Figure 11.15. In the two aggressive groups approximately 60% had a decrease or no change in CIMT and the outcomes were almost identical in the two subgroups treated with or without ezetimibe, however 61% of the standard group had an increase in CIMT.

ARBITER 6-HALTS [89] compared the effects of the addition of either nicotinic acid (niacin), as ERN, or ezetimibe to ongoing statin treatment of patients with a high-risk for clinical atherosclerosis. The patients had

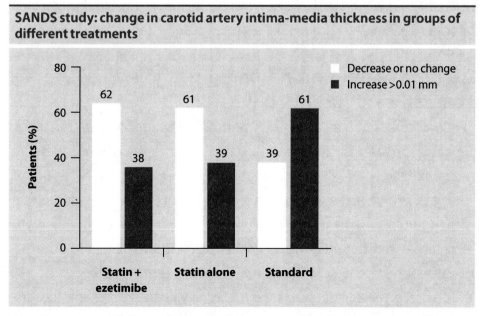

Figure 11.15 SANDS study: change in carotid artery intima-media thickness in groups of different treatments. Data from [88].

either a manifestation of clinical atherosclerosis or a CHD risk equivalent (including diabetes). All were on statin monotherapy, the men had a LDL-C 2.6 mmol/L (<100 mg/dL) and a HDL-C 1.3 mmol/L (<50 mg/dL) and the women 1.4 mmol/L (55 mg/dL). They were randomised for the administration of the additional treatment of open-label ezetimibe 10 mg/day or ERN, target dose 2000 mg/day. The primary endpoint was CIMT after 14 months, a secondary endpoint was a major cardiovascular event. When 60% of the planned sample size had completed the study the independent data advisory committee recommended that the trial should be stopped due to potentially paradoxical effects of ezetimibe as measured in terms of the primary endpoint. Total endpoint data from 208 patients was available and can be summarised as follows. Figure 11.16 shows the lipid results with the effect of niacin clearly raising HDL-C while in contrast, ezetimibe tended to slightly lower it. Likewise niacin, compared to ezetimibe, had a markedly better effect by lowering triglyceride levels, while ezetimibe was better than niacin at lowering LDL-C. The effects on CIMT are shown in Figure 11.17. In the niacin group CIMT decreased significantly over time while there were no changes in CIMT when treated with ezetimibe. Of further importance is that the incidence of clinical atherosclerosis was lower in the niacin group than in the ezetimibe group, 1% vs 5% ($p=0.04$). A major conclusion of the ARBITER trial was that niacin caused regression of CIMT and that it was superior to ezetimibe with regard to the effect on clinical atherosclerosis.

Addition of lipid-modifying drugs to statin treatment – ongoing trials

It is now well established that the treatment of patients at high risk for clinical arthrosclerosis with statins will reduce the rate of clinical events by approximately 25–40%. This implies, however, that manifestations of clinical atherosclerosis could not be prevented in 60–75% of such subjects by the treatment with statins alone, a figure that is unacceptably high. Therefore two different ways have been tried in the efforts to improve this situation by intensifying the lipid modification either by:

• further increasing the LDL lowering, e.g. by addition of ezetimibe, or
• raising the levels of the protective HDL, by the combination with niacin.

The further lowering of LDL

The addition of ezetimibe to statin treatment in lipid management further reduces already decreased LDL-C levels. However, what is not clear at present is the effect of this combined treatment on clinical atherosclerosis as is evident from the results of the three trials utilising the combined treatment of statin plus ezetimibe summarised in the sections above. Questions have been raised as to whether there is a beneficial effect of

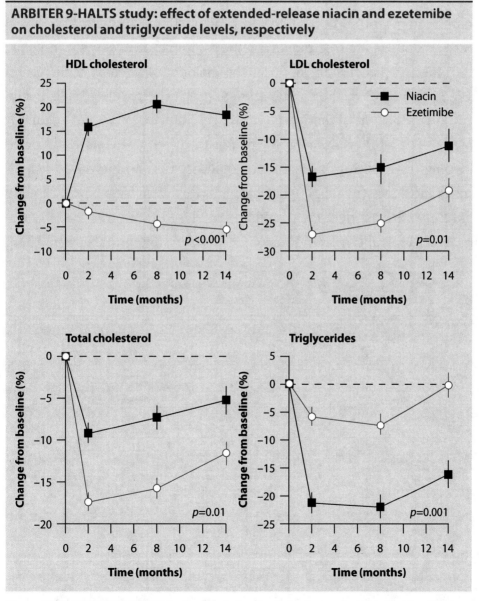

ARBITER 9-HALTS study: effect of extended-release niacin and ezetemibe on cholesterol and triglyceride levels, respectively

Figure 11.16 ARBITER 9-HALTS study: effect of extended-release niacin and ezetemibe on cholesterol and triglyceride levels, respectively. P-values are given for the comparison between the two groups at month 14. Data are for patients who completed the study (n=208). HDL, high-density lipoprotein; LDL, low-density lipoprotein. Data from [89].

treatment with the addition of ezetimibe that one might expect from the LDL-C mantra 'the lower the better'. However, there are two ongoing clinical studies with ezetimibe, SHARP is a trial of patients with renal failure and IMPROVE-IT compares the effects of simvastatin plus ezetimibe with simvastatin alone on hard endpoints in patients with acute coronary syndrome. The results of these two studies will soon be available and their size and hard endpoints will facilitate the judgement of effects of ezetimibe on the occurrence of clinical atherosclerosis. Of note is that in the recent SEAS trial [90] in which patients with aortic stenosis were randomised to treatment with the combination of simvastatin plus ezetimibe or placebo. In this trial the incident of cancers occurred in 105 and 70 cases in the combination and placebo groups, respectively ($p=0.01$) which the authors hypothesised might have been due to chance. In fact, a careful analysis performed at University of Oxford on large ongoing trials with this treatment could not find an increased risk of cancer incidence ($p=0.61$) [91]. However, when data from SEAS, SHARP and IMPROVE-IT were combined and analysed there was an increase in cancer mortality risk in the combined ezetimibe groups ($p=0.007$).

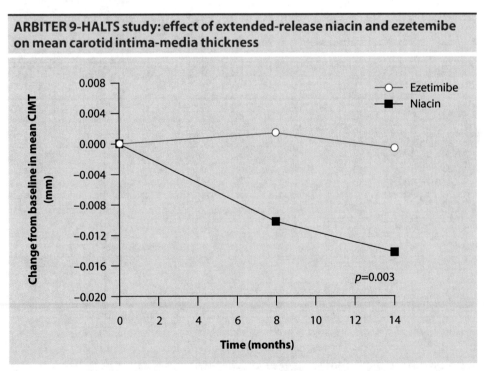

ARBITER 9-HALTS study: effect of extended-release niacin and ezetemibe on mean carotid intima-media thickness

Figure 11.17 **ARBITER 9-HALTS study: effect of extended-release niacin and ezetemibe on mean carotid intima-media thickness (CIMT).** Data from [89].

However, for statistical reasons the Oxford statisticians and epidemiologists believe that these mortality data are due entirely to chance rather than reflecting a true increase in cancer mortality.

Nevertheless the clinical results of SHARP and IMPROVE-IT will be of extreme importance with regard to the clinical effects of the combined treatment of statin plus ezetimibe on both clinical atherosclerosis and adverse effects.

The raising of HDL

Addition of nicotinic acid to statin treatment in lipid management raises HDL quite dramatically as shown in Figure 11.10. Two ongoing trials, AIM-HIGH and HPS2-THRIVE, will evaluate the effect of addition of niacin to statin treatment on outcomes of clinical atherosclerosis.

AIM-HIGH is a secondary prevention trial of patients with atherogenic dyslipidaemia (low HDL, high triglycerides) randomised to treatment with either simvastatin alone or simvastatin plus niacin for 3–5 years. Manifestations of clinical atherosclerosis are the primary endpoints. According to plans AIM-HIGH will be finished by September 2012.

HPS2-THRIVE, a secondary prevention study, will compare the effects of statin plus either placebo or MK-0524A (niacin with laropiprant [see above and Figure 11.12]) on cardiovascular events. This trial is due to report in 2013.

Chapter 12

Diabetic dyslipidaemia

In diabetes, dyslipidaemia was discovered long before hyperglycaemia. Berzelius, the inventor of the chemical formula notation now in use for over 200 years, and the founder of the Karolinska Institute, wrote in his biochemistry textbook in 1806 [92] '...*in diabetes one has much endeavoured to find urine sugar in the blood without success ... but has found so much fat that the plasma looked like an emulsion and deposited cream*'.

Today, 200 years later, when we can routinely determine blood glucose and glycated haemoglobin (HbA1c), it is well known that the major characteristics of the diabetic dyslipidaemia which is often called the lipid triad, consist of:
- hypertriglyceridaemia
- low concentrations of HDL
- abundance of small dense LDL

Additional components of diabetic dyslipidaemia are:
- increase of small dense HDL
- high levels of apoB
- low levels of apoA
- postprandial hyperlipidaemia

All components of the diabetic dyslipidaemia are tightly coupled metabolically to each other and the dyslipidaemia starts with a hepatic overproduction of triglyceride-rich lipoproteins (large VLDL particles). Of note is that LDL-C is often within normal limits in diabetics.

Clinical atherosclerosis and type 2 diabetes

There is strong epidemiological evidence of an independent association between diabetes and premature clinical atherosclerosis. The risk of developing clinical atherosclerosis manifestations for a patient with type 2 diabetes without evidence of any clinical atherosclerosis is equally high as for a non-diabetic who already has clinical atherosclerosis, which is why ATP III classifies diabetes in parallel with clinical atherosclerosis as a CHD risk equivalent (see Chapter 5).

Both type 1 and type 2 diabetes are associated with an increased risk of clinical atherosclerosis, such as CHD, cerebrovascular disease and peripheral vascular disease. Diabetes is a particularly strong risk factor in women and reduces the usual protection of women against clinical atherosclerosis

Management of the diabetic dyslipidaemia

Also for the treatment of the diabetic dyslipidaemia a healthy lifestyle, as discussed above in Chapter 10, is the basic keystone. It is of paramount importance to obtain blood glucose levels as normal as possible with a fasting blood glucose <6 mmol/L (108 mg/dL) and glycated haemoglobin (HbA1c) <7%. If these goals are not achieved by TLC, oral hypoglycaemic drugs should be added.

American Diabetes Association goals for lipids in diabetics	
Lipid goals	
LDL-C	
Without overt CVD	<2.6 mmol/L (<100 mg/dL)
With overt CVD*	<1.8 mmol/L (<70 mg/dL)
Triglycerides	<1.7 mmol/L (<150 mg/dL)
HDL-C*	
Men	>1.15 mmol/L (>40 mg/dL)
Women	>1.30 mmol/L (>50 mg/dL)
Management strategies	
In patients without overt CVD: <ul><li>age >40 years: LDL reduction of 30–40% by statin treatment</li><li>age <40 years and with other CVD risk factors: pharmacotherapy is appropriate if lifestyle changes fail to reach goals</li></ul>	
In patients with overt CVD: <ul><li>LDL reduction of 30–40% by statin treatment regardless of baseline lipid values</li></ul>	

Figure 12.1 American Diabetes Association goals for lipids in diabetics. *Optional. CVD, cardiovascular disease; HDL-C, high-density lipoprotein cholesterol; LDL-C, low-density lipoprotein cholesterol. Data from [93].

Lipid goals and pharmacological treatment

The lipid goals for the treatment of diabetic dyslipidaemia given by the American Diabetes Association (ADA) are shown in Figure 12.1. The LDL-C goals are identical to those recommended by ATP III, of note is that well-defined goals are presented for both triglycerides and HDL-C by ADA. If the goals for LDL-C are not achieved by TLC and good glycaemic control pharmacological treatment with lipid-modifying drugs has to be considered. Statins are the first-line choice, the recommendations for statin treatment in diabetic patients with or without CVD given by the ADA are shown in Figure 12.1. If statins for some reason, e.g. intolerance, exceptional dyslipidaemias or otherwise will not be the first-line lipid treatment the lipid regulating treatment should be prescribed with regard to the patient's lipid abnormality as recommended in Figures 10.2 and 10.3.

Effects of lipid management in diabetes on clinical atherosclerosis

Studies comprising diabetic subgroups

Several of the landmark trials with statins (see Chapter 8) had an sufficient number of patients with diabetes to allow post-hoc analysis of the effects in diabetes. The first of these, the 4S trial, provided evidence that lowering cholesterol with statins reduced the occurrence of cardiovascular events in patients with type 2 diabetes. For example in the 4S trial out of the 4444 patients 202 had diabetes with typical diabetic dyslipidaemia. During this five-year trial the incidence of major events of clinical atherosclerosis was 27% and 45%, respectively in placebo-treated patients with or without diabetes. Corresponding figures for the simvastatin treated patients were 19% and 23%, respectively. Statin treatment had thus reduced the incidence of clinical atherosclerosis in the diabetic subjects by nearly 50%. The large HPS included almost 6000 diabetic subjects. After five years of treatment with simvastatin major cardiovascular events had been reduced by 22% in the statin-treated diabetic patients compared with the placebo group. For the diabetic patients without evidence of clinical atherosclerosis at baseline there was a 33% reduction in CHD events as a result of the statin treatment.

Studies specific to diabetes

Four large studies on the clinical effect of lipid management on cardiovascular outcomes were performed in patients with diabetes: DAIS [79], CARDS [40], FIELD [81] and ACCORD [94]. In the DAIS trial 400 subjects with type 2 diabetes and good glycaemic control (HbA1c 7.5%) were randomised to placebo or fenofibrate (200 mg/day) for 3 years. The effects of fenofibrate on the lipid profile were total-C -10%, triglycerides -28%, LDL-C -6% and HDL-C +8%. Lipid changes in the placebo group were not significant. The progression of CAD was reduced by 42% and the decrease of coronary artery lumen was reduced by 40%. The DAIS was not powered to evaluate clinical endpoints. Nevertheless the number of combined CHD endpoints were 38 and 50 in the fenofibrate and placebo groups, respectively.

The FIELD study comprised 3795 patients with type 2 diabetes randomised to placebo or fenofibrate (200 mg/day) for five years. The incidence of total cardiovascular events was significantly reduced by 11% by the active treatment. However, the primary endpoint (death from CHD or non-fatal myocardial infarction) was only insignificantly diminished by 11%. The evaluation of FIELD is complicated because there was an unfortunate increased prescription and use of statins in the placebo group. A post-hoc analysis of FIELD [95] suggested that dyslipidaemic diabetic patients with both elevation of triglycerides and low levels of HDL benefited from the fibrate treatment.

In CARDS nearly 3000 patients with type 2 diabetes were randomised to treatment with atorvastatin (10 mg/day) or placebo. The lipid effects were LDL-C -31%, triglycerides -18% and HDL-C -10% the corresponding figures in the placebo group were -3%, -2% and -13%, respectively. This trial was terminated after 3.9 years, earlier than planned, due to the beneficial effects of the statin treatment. Major cardiovascular events occurred in 127 and 83 patients in the placebo and atorvastatin groups, respectively, a significant 37% reduction by the active treatment. CHD events, stroke and revascularisation procedures were also significantly diminished. The mortality rate was lowered by 27% by atorvastatin.

One recently published trial, the multicentre ACCORD lipid trial, has evaluated the cardiovascular outcomes of the lipid-modifying treatment with the combination of fenofibrate and statins [94] in 5518 subjects with type 2 diabetes. The patients were after intensive glycaemic control treated with open label simvastatin, according to national guidelines, and then randomised to receive the addition of either placebo or fenofibrate (160 mg/day). The effects of fenofibrate on the lipid profile are shown in Figure 12.2. The major effect was a lowering of triglycerides from

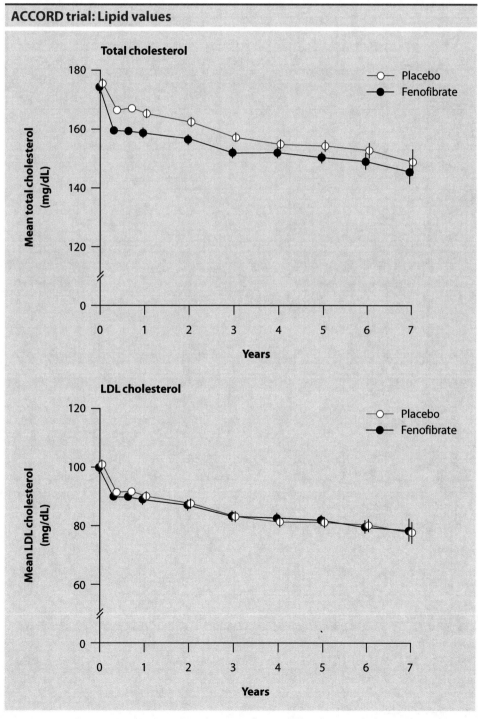

Figure 12.2 ACCORD trial: Lipid values (continues overleaf).

ACCORD trial: Lipid values (continued)

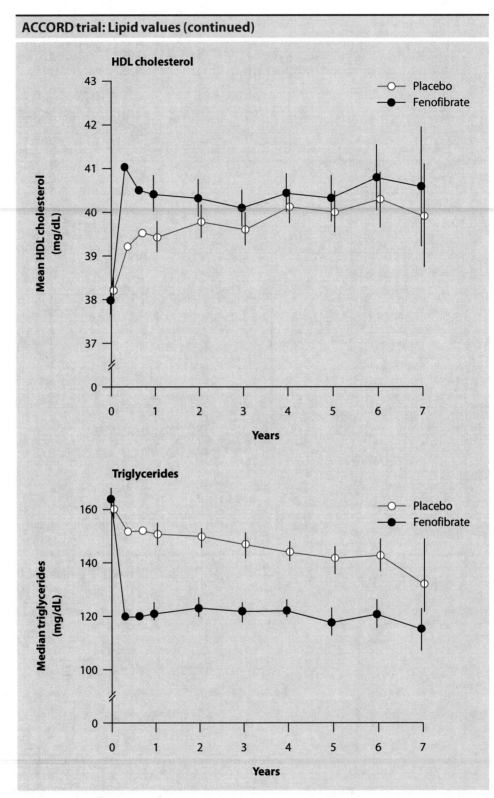

Figure 12.2 ACCORD trial: Lipid values (continued). Mean plasma levels of lipid parameters during the study. Bars represent 95% confidence intervals. P values for the differences between the two groups at the end of the study were 0.02, 0.16, 0.01 and 0.001 for Total-C, LDL-C, HDL-C and triglycerides, respectively [94].

1.89 mmol/L to 1.38 mmol/L (164 mg/dL to 122 mg/dL). LDL-C was not influenced in these statin-treated patients and HDL-C increased marginally. The annual rate of events of clinical atherosclerosis was 2.2% in the fenofibrate (with simvastatin) group and 2.4% in the placebo (with simvastatin) group, showing a non-significant difference ($p=0.32$). There was, however, a trend to beneficial effect on cardiovascular outcomes for diabetics with dyslipidaemia characterised by high triglycerides >2.3 mmol/L (>204 mg/dL) and low HDL-C <0.88 mmol/L (<34 mg/dL). In this group the primary outcome rate was 12.4% for those treated with fenofibrate vs 17.3% in the placebo group ($p=0.057$). These results suggesting a beneficial effect of fenofibrate on clinical atherosclerosis in dyslipidaemic diabetics are similar to those from post-hoc analysis in three previous fibrate trials: the HHS, the BIP trial and the FIELD study. Together the results of these four fibrate trials strongly suggest that fibrates not only effectively normalise the lipid profile of dyslipidaemic patients characterised by high triglycerides and low HDL levels but also reduces cardiovascular events in these high-risk dyslipidaemic patients, with and without diabetes.

Chapter 13

LDL apheresis

In severe hypercholesterolaemia as present in FH, particularly the rare homozygous form but also present in the much more common hetero-zygous forms, there may now and then be a need for more intensive cholesterol lowering than can be achieved by the combination of TLC and drugs. Plasma apheresis (from the Greek, to take away), particularly LDL apheresis, can then be a life saving cholesterol-lowering treatment for patients with severe hypercholesterolaemia resistant to lipid drugs.

In 1967 the clinical lipidologist De Gennes in Paris reported that treatment of a boy with homozygous FH with plasma apheresis every second day reduced plasma cholesterol from 18.6 mmol/L to 11.7 mmol/L (720 mg/dL to 450 mg/dL) [96], an excellent result at that time but totally insufficient cholesterol lowering according to today's guidelines.

Thompson and co-workers in London, UK, started systematic studies on the effects of plasma exchange in patients with homozygous FH in the 1970s [97] and demonstrated resolution of xanthomata as well as beneficial effects on aortic and coronary atherosclerosis in FH [98]. They also showed that apheresis resulted in improved survival rates of patients with severe hypercholesterolaemia [99].

The non-specific apheresis, in which whole plasma is removed and the remaining blood corpuscles are then transfused back into the patient, was developed into a specific LDL apheresis by Stoffel et al. in 1981 [100]. With this technique a specific removal of LDL and Lp(a) from the blood was achieved by adsorption of these apoB-containing lipoproteins from plasma on anti-LDL-Sepharose. Then the LDL-free plasma and the blood cells are returned to the patient. The rapid initial disappearance of LDL from plasma and the subsequent lowering of LDL-C over several days in response to LDL apheresis according to Stoffel is shown in Figure 13.1.

Beneficial effects on clinical atherosclerosis of LDL apheresis in FH has been reported in several trials. The largest and longest trial with LDL apheresis in patients with FH and CHD is the Japanese non-randomised Hokuriku study in which one group of patients (n=87) were aggressively treated with lipid-modifying drugs alone (a statin supplemented with other lipid drugs when needed) and the second group (n=43) treated with LDL apheresis as well for 6 years [101]; LDL cholesterol decreased by 28% and 58%, respectively in these two treatment groups. The number of coronary events was reduced by 70% by the LDL apheresis procedure compared to only aggressive medication (p <0.01, Figure 13.2).

Recommendations and guidelines for apheresis have been issued by several European countries and by the American Society for Apheresis. Recent recommendations on LDL apheresis is the HEART-UK guideline [102] which in summary says:

- The foremost indication for LDL apheresis (or plasma exchange) is the presence of homozygous FH which has not responded sufficiently well to drug therapy.
- In homozygotes where LDL-C has not been reduced by >50% and/ or to <9 mmol/L (350 mg/dL) apheresis should be started before age 7 years and performed weekly or bi-weekly and be combined with maximum dose of lipid drugs tolerated and most effective in the patient.
- In heterozygote FH the indications for LDL apheresis are less formal and rigid. Particular attention should be paid to heterozygotes with a bad family history for clinical atherosclerosis, progressive coronary disease and a LDL-C remaining >5 mmol/L (200 mg/dL).
- A further category that might be considered for LDL apheresis is for those with Lp(a) >1.5 mmol/L (>60 mg/dL).

The HEART-UK recommendations also describes in detail the five current methods for LDL apheresis with regard to equipment and procedures. All methods acutely decrease LDL-C by 50–75% with similar reductions in Lp(a). Interval means reductions of LDL-C vary between 45–55%.

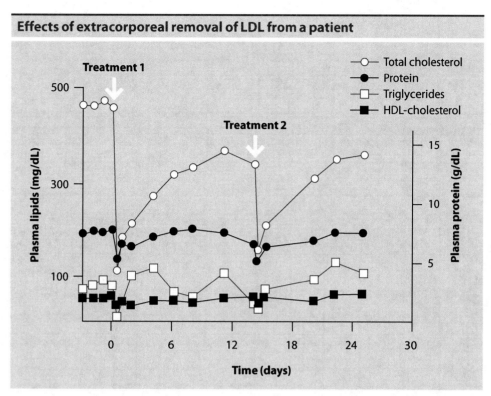

Figure 13.1 **Effects of extracorporeal removal of LDL from a patient.** HDL, high-density lipoprotein. Data from [100].

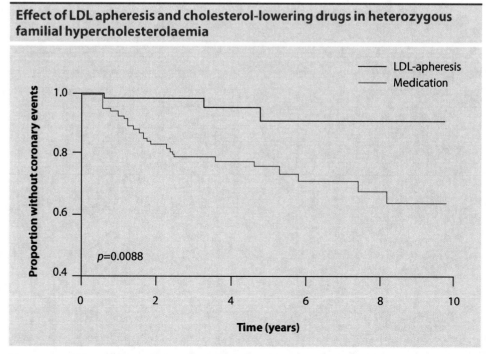

Figure 13.2 **Effect of LDL apheresis and cholesterol-lowering drugs in heterozygous familial hypercholesterolaemia:** Kaplan-Meier curves due for coronary events. LDL, low-density lipoprotein. Data from [101].

Chapter 14

Lipid-modifying agents under development

There are now several agents tailored for improving dyslipidaemic lipid profiles that have passed the preclinical testing and are presently in clinical trials. The two major fields for these new lipid drugs are:

1. To lower the levels of apoB-containing (atherogenic) lipoproteins, i.e. LDL, VLDL and Lp(a).
2. To increase the levels of apoA-containing (protective) lipoproteins, i.e. HDL.

Drugs for lowering apoB-containing lipoproteins

There is absolutely no doubt that statins are the first-line of choice of drugs for reducing the levels of LDL. Depending on type and dose of statin the lowering of LDL-C varies between 30–60% with intensive statin treatment. For most patients there is an excellent and sufficient LDL response with monotherapy with statins as is evident from Chapter 11. There are, however, some patients in need of more pronounced LDL lowering such as cases with severe FH or rapidly progressive clinical atherosclerosis for which nowadays statins are combined with other lipid drugs such as ezetimibe or niacin to obtain further reduction of LDL. Furthermore some 5-10% of patients are intolerant to statins, mainly due to myopathy adverse effects. For insufficient drug response, progressive clinical atherosclerosis and drug intolerance new effective LDL reducing drugs may find a place.

Inhibition of hepatic production of VLDL

The origin of the atherogenic apoB-containing lipoproteins is the hepatic production of VLDL particles which, after secretion into blood while still in blood, are converted to LDL particles of various sizes by different complex processes. To inhibit the production of VLDL would be an especially well-tailored treatment for patients for whom the capacity to remove LDL from blood is absent or reduced as for patients with homo- or heterozygous FH, respectively, where the LDL-receptor activity is absent or diminished. Two main points of attack are in use for lowering the production of VLDL by the liver:

- interference of the lipidation of the VLDL particles during their synthesis by slowing down this process by inhibition of the microsomal triglyceride transfer protein (MTP), and
- inhibition of the synthesis of apoB, the main structural part of the VLDL particles

Of note is that pronounced inhibition of hepatic VLDL formation by either mechanisms may cause accumulation of fat in the liver as a result of the reduced secretion of VLDL with its 'lipid cargo' from the liver.

Antisense inhibitor of apoB synthesis mipomersen

A recent 26-week phase 3 study in patients with homozygous hypercholesterolaemia on stable treatment with lipid-lowering drugs (statins, niacin etc or their combinations) were randomised to the addition of mipomersen 200 mg s.c. per week ($n=28$) or placebo ($n=17$) to their ongoing, continued lipid treatment [103]. Mean age was 31 years, baseline LDL-C/HDL-C were 11.4/1.0 (440/40 mg/dL) and 10.4/0.9 mmol/L (402/34 mg/dL) in the mipomersen and placebo groups, respectively.

Mipomersen lowered LDL-C by 25% down to 8.4 mmol/L (325 mg/dL; $p=0.0003$ vs placebo). The active treatment also reduced apoB and triglycerides by 27% and 17% but increased HDL-C by 15%. The time course for LDL-C, apoB and Lp(a) is shown in Figure 14.1.

MTP inhibitors lomitapide and implitapide

In a phase II study the MPT inhibitor lomitapide (AEGR 733) lowered LDL-C by 30% in monotherapy and by 46% in combination with ezetimibe,

Effect of mipomersen, an antisense inhibitor of apolipoprotein B synthesis, on lipid levels in homozygous familial hypercholesterolaemia

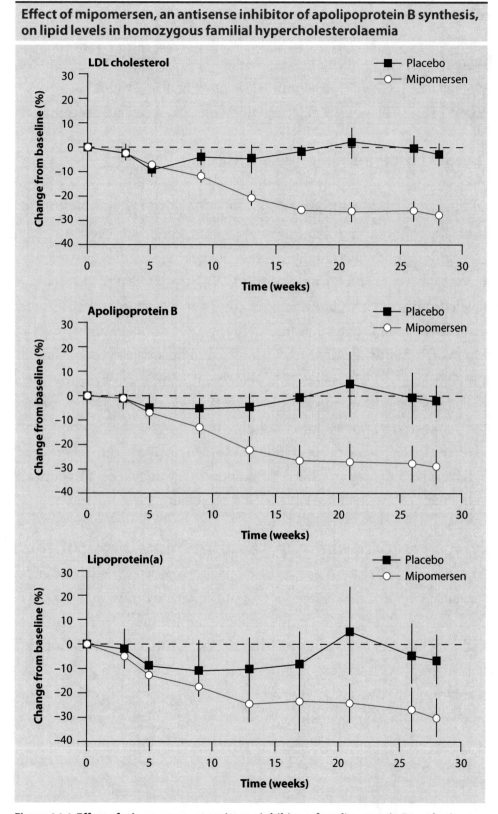

Figure 14.1 Effect of mipomersen, an antisense inhibitor of apolipoprotein B synthesis, on lipid levels in homozygous familial hypercholesterolaemia. Mipomersen is added to ongoing treatment with lipid-lowering drugs. Error bars indicate 95% confidence interval. LDL, low-density lipoprotein. Data from [103].

however, lomitapide was discontinued in 18% and 14%, respectively, due to elevations of transaminases and gastrointestinal adverse effects [104]. Similar results have been obtained with high doses of the MPT inhibitor implitapide (AEGR 427). The future development of MTP inhibitors will be to find doses giving sufficient lipid modification and acceptable safety profile.

Thyroid hormone analogue eprotirome

The long known clinical fact that hypo- and hyperthyroidism are associated respectively with hyper- and hypocholesterolaemia led to the discovery that that thyroxin lowers plasma cholesterol. Unfortunately the thyromimetic effects of thyroxin on the heart, including tachycardia, make thyroxin unsuitable as a routine lipid-lowering drug. The recently developed thyroid hormone analogue eprotirome, a molecule substituted with two bromide atoms, has minimal uptake in nonhepatic tissues but a high affinity for the lipid-lowering thyroid hormone receptor and is therefore subject to clinical testing. In a recent 12-week study eprotirome (0.1 mg/day) added to ongoing statin treatment lowered LDL-C, apoB, Lp(a) and triglycerides approximately 30% (Figure 14.2) without any adverse effects on the heart or bone [105]. Particularly the decrease of triglycerides and Lp(a) by this drug is noteworthy and more pronounced than the decrease monotherapy with statin causes.

Drugs for increasing apoA-containing lipoproteins

The reduction of risk for events of clinical atherosclerosis in high risk patients is approximately 25–40% by statin treatment with aggressive lowering of LDL-C. However, this implies that that new coronary events could not be prevented in 60–75% of subjects in high risk populations by monotherapy with statins, a figure which is unacceptably high. Because of this residual risk after lowering LDL it is necessary to find other strong lipid risk factors amenable for treatment to obtain better prevention of adverse events and their clinical complications, not forgetting the importance of non-lipid risk factors.

Low levels of HDL are as well as high levels of LDL well recognised as an important, independent lipid risk factor. The first identification of low values of HDL as a significant risk factor for CHD by the Miller brothers in the 1970s [106] has then been confirmed in a number of case-control as well as prospective studies. Results from epidemiological studies have suggested that there is a 2–3% decrease in cardiovascular risk for every 1 mg (0.03 mmol) increase in plasma HDL-C [107]. Therefore raising HDL by effective drugs in combination with LDL lowering with statin treatment may be a promising strategy for improved prevention of clinical atherosclerosis in high-risk patients.

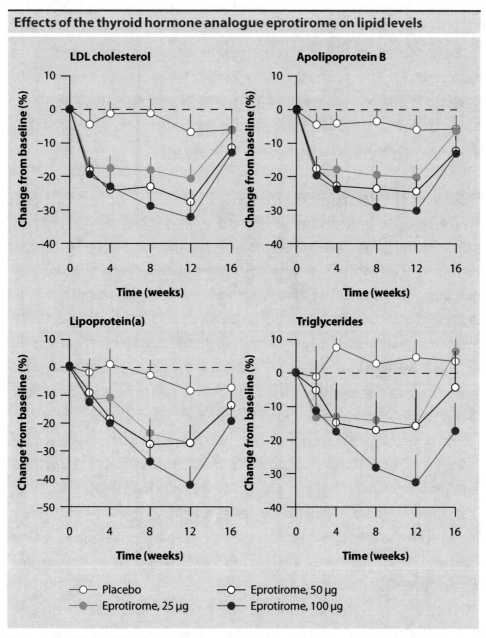

Figure 14.2 Effects of the thyroid hormone analogue eprotirome on lipid levels.
LDL, low-density lipoprotein. Bars represent 95% confidence interval. Data from [105].

Several factors influence HDL levels. Females have in general higher levels of HDL-C and lower levels of triglycerides than men. Low HDL can be caused by diabetes, metabolic syndrome, overweight, physical inactivity, smoking, β-blockers and certain genetic dyslipidaemias. There is a strong negative relation between the plasma concentrations of triglycerides and HDL, i.e. the higher concentration of triglycerides, the lower concentration of HDL. ATP III defines low HDL-C levels as <1.0 mmol/L (<40 mg/dL) for men and <1.3 mmol/L (<50 mg/dL) for women, and high triglycerides as values >1.7 mmol/L (>150 mg/dL).

Lipid-modifying drugs like statins, fibrates, bile acid sequestrants and ezetimibe may raise HDL-C by 5–15% while nicotinic acid has a much more pronounced effect on HDL with increases of approximately 20–40%, dose dependent. Of the new drugs raising HDL, inhibitors of CETP has recently attracted considerable interest.

Cholesteryl ester transfer protein

HDL is regulated by genetic as well as environmental factors. Cholesteryl ester transfer protein (CETP) is one of the important genetic factors for this regulation and acts as a key player in cholesterol transport by mediating the transfer of cholesteryl esters from HDL to VLDL/LDL and triglycerides from these lipoproteins to HDL. This action of CETP diminishes the cholesterol content of HDL and increases its triglyceride content. The hepatic clearance of the apoB lipoproteins enriched with cholesterol through the action of CETP will increase the elimination of cholesterol from peripheral tissues of the body via the bile.

The first clinical reports on the association between low CETP activity and high levels of HDL came from observations in Japanese families with genetic CETP deficiency and increased HDL levels [108]. Homozygotes with CETP deficiency have dramatically raised HDL levels and in addition low concentrations of LDL. It has been suggested that a deficiency of CETP with high levels of HDL may be protective for clinical atherosclerosis.

The first large clinical trial with an inhibitor to CETP, torcetrapib (ILLUMINATE, n=15,000) designed for testing the hypothesis that this drug, increasing HDL, might decrease the risk of events of clinical atherosclerosis. High-risk patients were randomised to treatment with either torcetrapib plus atorvastatin or atorvastatin-only [109]. Unexpectedly ILLUMINATE had to be stopped prematurely due to an increased occurrence of death and cardiac events in patients allocated to torcetrapib plus atorvastatin compared to patients treated with atorvastatin-only (hazard ratio 1.25, $p=0.001$) [109]. However, as expected torcetrapib increased HDL-C approximately 70% and lowered LDL-C by 25%.

The reasons for the harmful effects of torcetrapib have been much discussed. The authors of ILLUMINATE have reported several observations that might have contributed. The torcetrapib group compared to the control group had an increase of systolic blood pressure by 5.4 mmHg, from baseline compared to 0.9 mmHg in the atorvastatin-only group ($p <0.001$), a decrease in serum potassium, and increases of serum sodium and bicarbonate as well as aldosterone, changes consistent with hyperaldosteronaemia.

The results of the ILLUMINATE trial have raised questions such as 'The failure of torcetrapib: was it the molecule or the mechanism?' [110] and 'Is this the end of the road for CETP inhibitors after torcetrapib?' [111]. In the discussions it was suggested that the deleterious effects might be due to a torcetrapib-specific off-target effect and not an effect of the CETP-inhibition. Recently results of trials with two new CETP inhibitors anacetrapib [110] and dalcetrapib [113] were published.

The anacetrapib trial comprised 600 dyslipidaemic subjects randomised to two groups, one given 20 mg of atorvastatin and the other not given atorvastatin during 8 weeks. In addition, both groups had five subgroups treated with, respectively, placebo and anacetrapib at doses 10, 40, 150 and 300 mg daily (see Figure 14.3). Anacetrapib raised HDL-C significantly in a dose-dependent way from 10 to 150 mg but further increase to 300 mg did not cause a further increase (Figure 14.3). Maximal increase was approximately 120%. The effects on HDL-C in monotherapy and in combination with atorvastatin were equal. Anacetrapib in monotherapy lowered LDL-C also in a dose-dependent way, maximum lowering was approximately 40%, equal for 150 and 300 mg doses (Figure 14.4). The combined therapy with anacetrapib plus atorvastatin caused a still greater lowering of LDL-C up to 65% (Figure 14.4).

Because of the blood pressure increase observed with torcetrapib careful blood pressure monitoring was undertaken with six measurements 2 minutes apart, discarding the first measurement and averaging the other five. After 8 weeks of treatment there was no discernible effect of anacetrapib on either systolic or diastolic pressure.

The dalcetrapib trial comprised 135 participants with CHD or equivalent. During a run-in, pre-randomisation phase they were treated with atorvastatin. Those who achieved a LDL-C <2.6 mmol/L (<100 mg/dL) continued with atorvastatin and were in addition randomised to

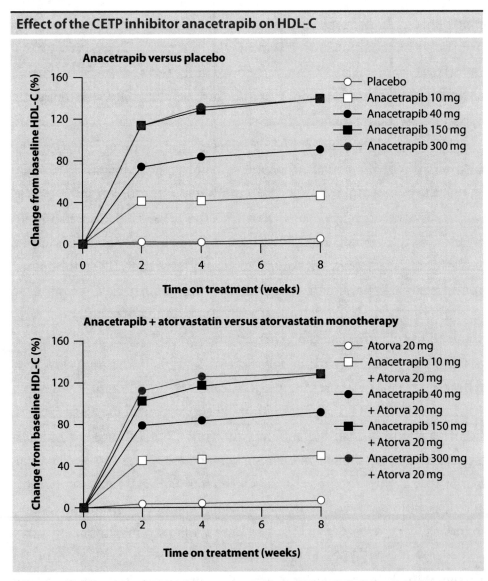

Figure 14.3 Effect of the CETP inhibitor anacetrapib on HDL-C. C, cholesterol; CETP, cholesteryl ester transfer protein; HDL, high-density lipoprotein. Data from [112].

treatment with either placebo or 900 mg of dalcetrapib daily for 24 plus 24 weeks. HDL-C increased by 33% in the dalcetrapib group and 3–4% in the placebo group. There was no additional lowering of LDL-C by dalcetrapib. The treatment with dalcetrapib did not affect blood pressures.

A very recent article has reported on the safety and lipid effects of the new CETP inhibitor anacetrapib in patients with CHD or at CHD risk [114]. Altogether 1623 patients, taking a statin, having LDL-C between 1.3–2.6 mmol/L (50–100 mg/dL and HDL-C <1.6 mmol/L (<60 mg/dL), ages 18–80 years were included in this trial. They had

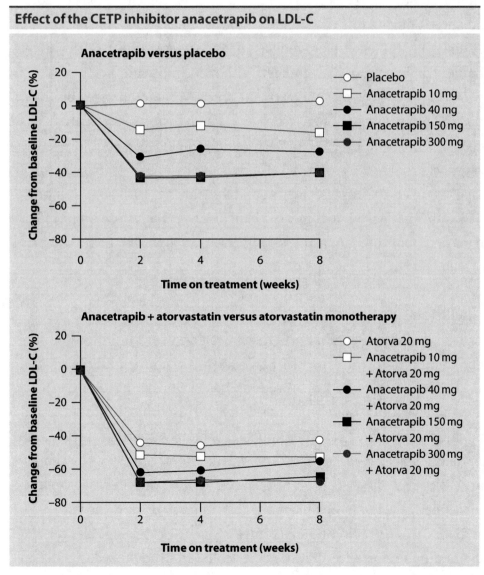

Figure 14.4 Effect of the CETP inhibitor anacetrapib on LDL-C. C, cholesterol; CETP, cholesteryl ester transfer protein; LDL, low-density lipoprotein. Data from [112].

evidence of CHD or were at high risk for CHD (Framingham risk score >20%). Patients were randomised double blind to placebo or anacetrapib 200 mg once daily. They were instructed to continue ongoing lipid modifying therapy.

Figure 14.5 shows the almost constant levels during the study of LDL-C and HDL-C in the placebo group as well as in the treatment group after the initial response to active treatment. On average LDL-C was reduced by 40% and HDL-C raised by nearly 140% by the addition of anacetrapib to statin in accordance with previous trials with anacetrapib (see above). As expected the changes in concentrations of apoB and apoA-1 during this trial followed those of LDL-C and HDL-C levels. In addition Lp(a) levels were reduced by 35% in this study, a drug effect of anacetrapib previously only seen with nicotinic acid.

During the 76 weeks of treatment there were no changes in blood pressure, electrolytes or aldosterone levels with anacetrapib treatment as was the case with the earlier CETP inhibitor torcetrapib. Cardiovascular events occurred in 2.6% and 2.0% in the placebo and anacetrapib group, respectively (p=0.40). In conclusion, it is clear that the CETP inhibitor anacetrapib has a well-documented beneficial anti-atherosclerotic effect on plasma lipids in man by increasing HDL and lowering LDL and Lp(a) without causing any major side-effects.

Conclusion

The trials with CETP inhibitors in man have given varying clinical results depending on type of drug. All have, however, consistently increased the concentration of HDL-C. Torcetrapib caused severe adverse effects with increased mortality and morbidity. It raised blood pressure and appeared to stimulate to hyperaldosteronaemia. Neither anacetrapib nor dalcetrapib increased mortality and morbidity or raised blood pressures. Anacetrapib appeared to increase HDL-C and decrease LDL-C most effectively. From the lipid management point of view the two CETP inhibitors, anacetrapib and dalcetrapib appear promising. It is now of outstanding importance that they are tested in randomised, long-term clinical studies with regard to their effects on outcomes of events of clinical atherosclerosis, safety and adverse effects.

Lipid management tomorrow

It is very tempting indeed to believe and hope that combined lipid management which at the same time raises HDL and lowers LDL will reduce the risk of manifestations of clinical atherosclerosis for high-risk patients. Today the best combination to obtain this goal is a treatment with statin plus nicotinic acid. Tomorrow it may also be a statin plus an inhibitor of CETP.

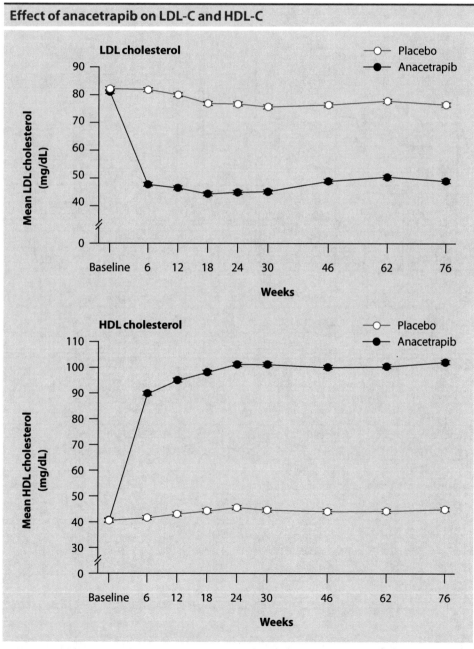

Figure 14.5 Effect of anacetrapib on LDL-C and HDL-C. Mean values for LDL-C and HDL-C during the study. HDL-C, high-density lipoprotein cholesterol; LDL-C, low-density lipoprotein cholesterol. Reproduced with permission from [114].

References

1   Murray CJL, Lopez AD (eds). *The global burden of disease: a comprehensive assessment of mortality and disability from diseases, injuries, and risk factors in 1990 and projected to 2020.* Boston, USA: Harvard School of Public Health, 1996.

2   World Health Statistics. Cause-specific mortality and morbidity. World Health Organization, 2009. Available at www.who.int/whosis/whostat/2009/en/index.html. [Last accessed 9 February 2011].

3   Hansson GK. Atherosclerosis – an immune disease. The Anitschkov lecture 2007. Atherosclerosis 2009;202:2–10.

4   Doyle JT. Risk factors in coronary heart disease. NY State J Med 1963;May:1317–1320.

5   Kannel WB, Dawber TR, Kagan A, et al. Factors of risk in the development of coronary heart disease– Six year follow-up experience. The Framingham Study. Ann Int Med 1961;55:33–50.

6   Yusuf S, Hawken S, Ounpuu S, et al. Effect of potentially modifiable risk factors associated with myocardial infarction in 52 countries (the INTERHEART study): case-control study. Lancet 2004;364:937–952.

7   McQueen MJ, Hawken S, Wang X, et al. Lipids, lipoproteins, and apolipoproteins as risk markers of myocardial infarction in 52 countries (the INTERHEART study): a case-control study. Lancet 2008;372:224–233.

8   Beaumont JL, Carlson LA, Cooper GR, et al. Classification of hyperlipidaemias. Bull WHO Health Org Mond Santé 1970;43:891–915.

9   National Cholesterol Education Program. Second Report of the Expert Panel on Detection,Valuation, and Treatment in Adults (Adult Treatment Panel II). Circulation 1994;89:1329–1445.

10 European guidelines on cardiovascular disease prevention in clinical practice: executive summary. Eur J Cardiovasc Prev Rehab 2007;14(Suppl 2):E1–E40.

11 Executive summary of the third report of the National cholesterol Education Program (NCEP) expert panel on detection, evaluation, and treatment of high blood cholesterol in adults (Adult Treatment Panel III, ATP III). JAMA 2001;285:2486–2497.

12 Implications of recent clinical trials for the National Cholesterol Education Program Adult Treatment Panel III Guidelines. Circulation 2004;110:227–239.

13 Walldius G, Jungner I, Holme I, et al. High apolipoprotein B, low apolipoprotein A-I, and improvement in the prediction of fatal myocardial infarction (AMORIS study): a prospective study. Lancet 2001;358:2026–2033.

14 Kannel WB, Castelli WP, Gordon T, et al. Serum cholesterol, lipoproteins, and the risk of coronary heart disease: the Framingham Study. Ann Intern Med 1971;74:1–12.

15 Wilson PWF, Castelli WP, Kannel WB. Coronary risk prediction in adults: the Framingham heart study. Am J Cardiol 1987;59(G):91–94.

16 Wilson PWF. Risk scores for prediction of coronary heart disease: an update. Endocrinol Metab Clin N Am 2009;38:33–34.

17 Wilson PW, D'Agostino RB, Levy D, et al. Prediction of coronary heart disease using risk factor categories. Circulation 1998;97:1837–1847.

18 Assmann G, Cullen P, Schulte H. Simple scoring scheme for calculating the risk of acute coronary events based on the 10-year follow-up of the prospective cardiovascular Münster (PROCAM) study. Circulation 2002;105(3):310–315.

19 Conroy RM, Pyorala K, Fitzgerald AP, et al. Estimation of ten-year risk of fatal cardiovascular disease in Europe: the SCORE project. Eur Heart J 2003;24:987–1003.

20 Ridker PM, Rifai N, Cook NR, et al. Non-HDL cholesterol, apolipoprotein A-I and B100, standard lipid measures, lipid ratios, and CRP as risk factors for cardiovascular disease in women. JAMA 2005;294:326–333.

21 Ingelsson E, Schaefer EJ, Contois JH, et al. Clinical utility of different lipid measures for prediction of coronary heart disease in men and women. JAMA 2007;298:776–785.

22 Walldius G, Jungner I, Aastveit AH, et al. The apoB/apoA-I ratio is better than the cholesterol ratios to estimate the balance betweenplasma prostherogenic and antiatherogenic lipoproteins and to predict coronary risk. Clin Chem Lab Med 2004;42:1355–1363.

23 Durrington P, Sniderman A. *Fast Facts – Hyperlipidemia, 3rd edition*. Oxford, UK: Health Press, 2008.

24 Lipid Clinics Research Program. The Lipid Research Clinics Coronary Primary Prevention Trial results. I. Reduction in incidence of coronary artery disease. II. The relationship of reduction in incidence of coronary heart disease to cholesterol lowering. JAMA 1984;251:351–374.

25 The Scandinavian Simvastatin Survival Study Group. Randomized trial of cholesterol lowering in 4444 patients with coronary heart disease: the Scandinavian Simvastatin Survival Study (4S). Lancet 1994;344:1383–1389.

26 Sacks FM, Pfeffer MA, Moyé LA, et al; Cholesterol and Recurrent Events Trial Investigators. The effect of pravastatin on coronary events after myocardial infarction in patients with average cholesterol levels. N Engl J Med 1996;335:1001–1009.

27 The Long-term Intervention with Pravastatin in Ischaemic Disease (LIPID) Study Group. Prevention of cardiovascular events and death with pravastatin in patients with coronary heart disease and a broad range of initial cholesterol levels. N Engl J Med 1998;339:1349–1357.

28 Shepherd J, Cobbe SM, Ford I, et al; West of Scotland Coronary Prevention Study Group. Prevention of coronary heart disease with pravastatin in men with hypercholesterolemia. N Engl J Med 1995;333:1301–1307.

29 Downs JR, Clearfield M, Weis S, et al. Primary prevention of acute coronary events with lovastatin in men and women with average cholesterol levels: results of AFCAPS/TexCAPS. Air Force/Texas Coronary Atherosclerosis Prevention Study. JAMA 1998;279:1615–1622.

30 Endo A, Kuroda M, Tanzawa K. Competitive inhibition of 3-hydroxy-methylglutaryl coenzyme A reductase by ML-236A and ML-236B fungal metabolites, having hypocholesterolemic activity. FEBS Lett 1976;72:323–326.

31 Yamamoto A, Sudo H, Endo A. Therapeutic effects of ML-236B in primary hypercholesterolemia. Atherosclerosis 1980;35:259–266.

32 Heart Protection Study Collaborative Group. MRC/BHF Heart Protection Study of cholesterol lowering with simvastatin in 20,536 high-risk individuals: a randomised placebo-controlled trial. Lancet 2002;360:7–22.

33 Holdaas H, Fellström B, Jardine AG, et al. for the ALERT Study Investigators. Effect of fluvastatin on cardiac outcomes in renal transplant recipients: a multicentre, randomised, placebo-controlled trial. Lancet 2003;361(9374):2024–2031.

34 ALLHAT Officers and Coordinators for the ALLHAT Collaborative Research Group. Major outcomes in moderately hypercholesterolemic, hypertensive patients randomized to pravastatin vs usual care: The Antihypertensive and Lipid-Lowering Treatment to Prevent Heart Attack Trial (ALLHAT-LLT). JAMA 2002;288(23):2998–3007.

35 Shepherd J, Blauw GJ, Murphy MB, et al. Pravastatin in elderly individuals at risk of vascular disease (PROSPER): a randomised controlled trial. Lancet 2002;360:1623–1630.

36 Sever PS, Dahlöf B, Poulter NR, et al. for the ASCOT Investigators. Prevention of coronary and stroke events with atorvastatin in hypertensive patients who have average or lower-than-average cholesterol concentrations, in the Anglo-Scandinavian Cardiac Outcomes Trial – Lipid Lowering Arm (ASCOT-LLA): a multicentre randomised controlled trial. Lancet 2003;361(9364):1149–1158.

37 Serruys PWJ, de Feyter P, Macaya C, et al. Fluvastatin for prevention of cardiac events following successful first percutaneous coronary intervention a randomized controlled trial. JAMA 2002;287:3215–3222.

38 Amarenco P, Bogousslavsky J, Callahan A 3rd, et al., SPARCL investigators. High-dose atorvastatin after stroke or transient ischemic attack. N Engl J Med 2006;355:549–559.

39 Colhoun HM, Betteridge DJ, Durrington PN, et al. Primary prevention of cardiovascular disease with atorvastatin in type 2 diabetes in the Collaborative Atorvastatin Diabetes Study (CARDS): multicentre randomised placebo-controlled trial. Lancet 2004;364:685–696.

40 Shepherd J, Cobbe SM, Ford I. et al. for the West of Scotland Coronary Prevention Study Group. Prevention of coronary heart disease with pravastatin in men with hypercholesterolemia. New Engl J Med 1995:333:1301–1307.

41 Gotto AM Jr, Whitney E, Stein EA, et al. Application of the National Cholesterol Education Program and joint European treatment criteria and clinical benefit in the Air Force/Texas Coronary Atherosclerosis Prevention Study (AFCAPS/TexCAPS). Eur Heart J 2000;21(19):1627–1633.

42 Mc Kenney JM, Ganz P, Wiggins BS, Saseen JS. Statins. In: *Clinical lipidology. A companion to Braunwald's Heart Disease*. Edited by CM Ballantyne. Philadelphia, USA: Saunders, 2009.

43 La Rosa JC, Grundy S, Waters D, et al. Intensive lipid lowering with atorvastatin in patients with stable coronary disease. N Engl J Med 2005;352:1425–1435.

44 Baigent C, Keech A, Kearney PM, et al. Efficacy and safety of cholesterol-lowering treatment: prospective meta-analysis of data from 90,056 participants in 14 randomised trials of statins. Lancet 2005;366:1267–1278.

45 Kizer JR, Madias C, Wilner B, et al. Relation of different measures of low-density lipoprotein cholesterol to risk of coronary artery disease and death in a meta-regression analysis of large-scale trials of statin therapy. Am J Cardiol 2010;105:1289–1296.

46 Wood DA, Wray R, Poulter N, et al. JDS2: Joint British Societies' guidelines on prevention of cardiovascular disease in clinical practice. Heart 2005;91(Suppl V):v1–52.

47 NICE Clinical guideline 67. Cardiovascular risk assessment and the modification of blood lipids for the primary and secondary prevention of cardiovascular disease. Available at www.nice.org.uk/cg67.

48 Jones PH, Davidson MH, Stein EA, et al. Comparison of the efficacy and safety of rosuvastatin versus atorvastatin, simvastatin, and pravastatin across doses (STELLAR trial). Am J Cardiol 2003;92:152–160.

49 Carlson LA. Nicotinic acid: the broad-spectrum lipid drug. A 50th anniversary review. J Int Med 2005;258:94–114.

50 The Coronary Drug Project Research Group. Clofibrate and niacin in coronary heart disease. JAMA 1975;231:360–381.

51 Brown BG. Niaspan® in the management of dyslipidaemia: the evidence. Eur Heart J Suppl 2006;8(suppl. F):F60-F67.

52 Brown BG, Canner PL, McGovern ME, et al. Nicotinic acid. In: *Clinical lipidology. A companion to Braunwald's Heart Disease*. Edited by CM Ballantyne. Philadelphia, USA: Saunders, 2009.

53 Carlson LA, Rosenhamer G. Reduction of mortality in the Stockholm ischaemic heart disease secondary prevention study by combined treatment with clofibrate and nicotinic acid. Acta Med Scand 1988;223:405–418.

54 Brown BG, Zhao X-Q, Chait A, et al. Simvastatin and niacin, antioxidant vitamins, or the combination for the prevention of coronary disease. N Engl J Med 2001;345:1583–1592.

55 Carlson LA, Hamsten A, Asplund A. Pronounced lowering of serum levels of lipoprotein Lp(a) in hyperlipidaemic subjects treated with nicotinic acid. J Intern Med 1989;226:271–276.

56 Sprecher DL. Raising high-density lipoprotein cholesterol with niacin and fibrates: A comparative review. Am J Cardiol 2000;86(suppl):46L–50L.

57 Xydakis AM, Ballantyne CM. Combination therapy for combined dyslipidemia. Am J Cardiol 2002;90(suppl):21K–29K.

58 Paolini JF, Mitchel YB, Reyes R, et al. Effects of laropiprant on nicotinic acid-induced flushing in patients with dyslipidemia. Am J Cardiol 2008;101:625–630.

59 Perry CM. Extended release niacin (nicotinic acid)/laropiprant. Drugs 2009;69(12):1665–1679.

60 Carlson LA. Niaspan, the prolonged (extended, ER) release preparation of nicotinic acid (niacin), the broad spectrum lipid drug. Int J Clin Practice 2004;58:706–713.

61 Thorp JM, Waring WS. Modification of metabolism and distribution of lipids by ethyl chlorophenoxyisobutyrate. Nature 1962;194:948–949.

62 Hellman L, Zumoff B, Kessler G, et al. Reduction of Cholesterol and Lipids in Man by Ethyl p-Chlorophenoxyisobutyrate. Ann Int Med 1963;59:477.

63 Barter PJ, Rye K-A. Cardioprotective properties of fibrates. Which fibrate, which patients, what mechanism? Circulation 2006;113:1533–1555.

64 Oliver MF, Heady JA, Morris JN, et al. WHO cooperative trial on primary prevention of ischaemic heart disease with clofibrate to lower serum cholesterol; final mortality follow-up. Lancet 1984;324(8403):600–604.

65 Frick MH, Elo O, Haapa K, et al. Helsinki Heart Study. primary prevention trial with gemfibrozil in middle-aged men with dyslipidaemia. Safety of treatment, changes in risk factors, and incidence of coronary heart disease. N Engl J Med 1987;317:1237–1245.

66 Rubins HB, Robins SJ, Collins D, et al; for the Veterans Aff airs High-Density Lipoprotein Cholesterol Intervention Trial Study Group. Gemfibrozil for the secondary prevention of coronary heart disease in men with low levels of high-density lipoprotein cholesterol. N Engl J Med 1999;341:410–418.

67 Jun M, Foote C, Lv J, et al. Effects of fibrates on cardiovascular outcomes: a systematic review and meta-analysis. Lancet 2010;375:1875–1884.

68 Arthur JB, Raffle RB, Ashby WR, et al. Trial of clofibrate in the treatment of ischaemic heart disease. Five-year study by a group of physicians of the Newcastle upon Tyne region. BMJ 1971;4:767–775.

69 Research Committee of the Scottish Society of Physicians. Ischaemic heart disease: a secondary prevention trial using clofibrate. Report by a research committee of the Scottish Society of Physicians. BMJ 1971;4:775–784.

70 The Veterans Administration Cooperative Study Group. The treatment of cerebrovascular disease with clofibrate. Final report of the Veterans Administration Cooperative Study of Atherosclerosis, Neurology Section. Stroke 1973;4:684–693.

71 WHO Cooperative Trial Committee of Principal Investigators. A co-operative trial in the primary prevention of ischaemic heart disease using clofibrate. Report from the Committee of Principal Investigators. Br Heart J 1978;40:1069–1118.

72 Hanefeld M, Fischer S, Schmechel H, et al. Diabetes Intervention Study. Multi-intervention trial in newly diagnosed NIDDM. Diabetes Care 1991;14:308–317.

73 Nilsson J, Ericsson CG, Hamsten A, et al. Bezafibrate following acute myocardial infarction: important findings from the Bezafibrate Coronary Atherosclerosis Intervention Trial. Fibrinolysis Proteolysis 1997;11(suppl 1):159–162.

74 Lipid Coronary Angiography Trial (LOCAT) Study Group. Frick MH, Syvanne M, Nieminen MS, et al. Prevention of the angiographic progression of coronary and vein-graft atherosclerosis by gemfibrozil after coronary bypass surgery in men with low levels of HDL cholesterol. Circulation 1997;96:2137–2143.

75 Elkeles RS, Diamond JR, Poulter C, et al. Cardiovascular outcomes in type 2 diabetes. A double-blind placebo-controlled study of bezafibrate: the St. Mary's, Ealing, Northwick Park Diabetes Cardiovascular Disease Prevention (SENDCAP) Study. Diabetes Care 1998;21:641–648.

76 The BIP Study Group. Secondary prevention by raising HDL cholesterol and reducing triglycerides in patients with coronary artery disease: the Bezafibrate Infarction Prevention (BIP) study. Circulation 2000;102:21–27.

77   Diabetes Atherosclerosis Intervention Study Investigators. Effect of fenofibrate on progression of coronary-artery disease in type 2 diabetes: the Diabetes Atherosclerosis Intervention Study, a randomised study. Lancet 2001;357:905–910.

78   Meade T, Zuhrie R, Cook C, et al. Bezafibrate in men with lower extremity arterial disease: randomised controlled trial. BMJ 2002;325:1139.

79   The FIELD study investigators. Effects of long-term fenofibrate therapy on cardiovascular events in 9795 people with type 2 diabetes mellitus (the FIELD study): randomised controlled trial. Lancet 2005;366:1849–1861.

80   Ginsberg HN, Elam MB, Lovato LC, et al; for the ACCORD Study Group. Effects of combination lipid therapy in type 2 diabetes mellitus. N Engl J Med 2010;362:1563–1574.

81   Otvos JD, Collins D, Freedman DS et al. Low-density lipoprotein and high-density lipoprotein particle subclasses predict coronary events and are favourably changed by gemfibrozil treatment in VA-HIT. Circulation 2006;113:1556–1563.

82   McCormack T, Harvey P, Gaunt R, et al. Incremental cholesterol reduction with ezetimibe/ simvastatin, atorvastatin and rosuvastatin in UK General Practice (IN-PRACTICE): a randomised controlled trial of achievement of Joint British Societies (JBS-2) cholesterol targets. Int J Clin Pract 2010;64(8):1006-1008.

83   Kastelein JJP, Akdim F, Stroes ESG, et al. Simvastatin with or without ezetimibe in familial hypercholesterolemia. N Engl J Med 2008;358;1431–1443.

84   Brown BG, Taylor AJ. Does ENHANCE diminish confidence in lowering LDL or in ezetimibe? N Engl J Med 2008;358(14):1504-1507.

85   American College of Cardiology. Statement from the American College of Cardiology Related to the ENHANCE Trial. 15 January 2008. Available at www.cardiosource.org/News-Media/Media-Center/News-Releases/2008/01/15.aspx. [Last accessed 9 February 2011].

86   Fleg JL, Mete M, Howard BV, et al. Effect of statins alone versus statins plus ezetimibe on carotid atherosclerosis in type 2 diabetes: The SANDS (Stop Atherosclerosis in Native Diabetics Study) trial. J Am Coll Cardiol 2008;52:2198–2205.

87   Taylor AJ, Villines TC, Stanek EJ, et al. Extended-release niacin or ezetimibe and carotid intima-media thickness. N Engl J Med 2009;361:2113–2122.

88   Rossebö AB, Pedersen TR, Boman K, et al. Intensive lipid lowering with simvastatin and ezetimibe in aortic stenosis. N Engl J Med 2008;359:1343–1356.

89   Peto R, Emberson J, Landray M, et al. Analyses of cancer data from three ezetimibe trials. N Engl J Med 2008;359:1357–1366.

90   Berzelius JJ. Föreläsningar i Djurkemien. Stockholm: Carl Delén, 1806.

91   American Diabetes Association. Standards of medical care in diabetes – 2006. Diabetes Care 2006;29(suppl 1):S4–S42.

92   The ACCORD Study Group. Effects of combination lipid therapy in type 2 diabetes mellitus. N Engl J Med 2010;362:1563–1574.

93   Scott R, O'Brien R, Fulcher G, et al. Effects of fenofibrate treatment on cardiovascular disease risk in 9795 people with type 2 diabetes and various components of the metabolic syndrome: the fenofibrate intervention and event lowering in diabetes (FIELD) study. Diabetes Care 2009;32:494–498.

94   De Gennes JL, Touraine R, Mannaud B, et al. Formes homozygotes cutanéo-tendineuses de xanthomatose hypercholestérolique dans une observation familiale exemplaire – essai de plasmaphérèse à titre de traitement heroic. Bull Soc Med Hop Paris 1967;118:1377–1380.

95   Thompson GR, Lowenthal R, Myant NB. Plasma exchange in the management of homozygous familial hypercholesterolaemia. Lancet 1975;305(7918):1208–1210.

96   Thompson GR, Myant NB, Kilpatrick D, et al. Assessment of long-term plasma exchange for familial hypercholesterolaemia. Brit Heart J 1980;43:680–688.

97   Thompson GR, Miller JP, Breslow JL. Improved survival of patients with homozygous hypercholesterolaemia treated with plasma exchange. BMJ 1985;291:1671–1673.

98 Stoffel W, Borberg H, Greve V, et al. Application of specific extracorporeal removal of low density lipoprotein in familial hypercholesterolaemia. Lancet 1981;2(8254):1005–1007.

99 Mabuchi H, Koizumi J, Shimizu M, et al. Long-term efficacy of low-density lipoprotein apheresis on coronary heart disease in familial hypercholesterolaemia. Am J Cardiol 1998;82:1495–1489.

100 GR Thompson, HEART-UK LDL Apheresis Working Group. Recommendations for the use of LDL apheresis. Atherosclerosis 2008;198:247–255.

101 Raal FJ, Santos RD, Blom DJ, et al. Mipomersen, an apolipoprotein B synthesis inhibitor, for lowering LDL cholesterol concentrations in patients with homozygous familial hypercholesterolaemia: a randomised, double-blind, placebo-controlled trial. Lancet 2010;375:998–1006.

102 Samaha FF, McKenney J, Bloedon LT, et al. Inhibition of microsomal triglyceride transfer protein alone or with ezetimibe in patients with moderate hypercholesterolemia. Nat Clin Pract Cardiovasc Med 2008;5:506–508.

103 Ladenson PW, Jens D, Kristensen MD, et al. Use of the thyroid hormone analogue Eprotirome in statin treated dyslipidemia. N Engl J Med 2010;362:906–916.

104 Miller GJ, Miller NE. Plasma high-density lipoprotein concentration and development of ischaemic heart-disease. Lancet 1975;305(7897):16–19.

105 Gordon DJ, Probstfield JL, Garrison RJ, et al. High-density lipoprotein cholesterol and cardiovascular disease. Four prospective American studies. Circulation 1989;79:8–15.

106 Brown ML, Inazu A, Hesler CB, et al. Molecular basis of lipid transfer protein deficiency in a family with increased high-density lipoprotein. Nature 1989;342:448–451.

107 Barter PJ, Caulfield M, Eriksson M, et al. Effects of torcetrapib in patients at high risk for coronary events. N Engl J Med 2007;357:2109–2192.

108 Tall AR, Yvan-Charvet L, Wang N, et al. The failure of torcetrapib: was it the molecule or the mechanism? Arterioscl Thromb Vasc Biol 2007;27:257–260.

109 Joy T, Hegele RA. The end of the road for CETP inhibitors after torcetrapib. Curr Opin Cardiol 2009;24:364–371.

110 Bloomfield D, Carlson GL, Sapre A, et al. Efficacy and safety of the cholesteryl ester transfer protein inhibitor anacetrapib as monotherapy and coadministered with atorvastatin in dyslipidemic patients. Am Heart J 2009;157:352–360.

111 Stein EA, Roth EM, Rhyne JM, et al. Safety and tolerability of dalcetrapib (RO4607381/JTT-705): results from a 48-week trial. Eur Heart J 2010;31:480–488.

112 Cannon PC, Shah S, Dansky HM, et al. Safety of anacetrapib in patients with or at high risk for coronary heart disease. New Engl J Med 2010;363:2406–2415.